HOUSE OFFICER SERIES

Case Studies in Emergency Medicine

HOUSE OFFICER SERIES

Case Studies in Emergency Medicine

Lidia Pousada, MD, FACP

Director, Geriatric Unit and Consult Service
Associate Director, Unified Division of Geriatrics
Montefiore Medical Center, Bronx, New York
Assistant Professor of Medicine
Albert Einstein College of Medicine, Bronx, New York

David B. Levy, DO

Attending Physician, Emergency Department
Allegheny General Hospital, Pittsburgh, Pennsylvania
Assistant Professor, Emergency Medicine
Medical College of Pennsylvania, Allegheny Campus
Pittsburgh, Pennsylvania

Harold H. Osborn, MD, FACEP, FACP, ABMT

Director of Research, Emergency Medicine Residency Training Program
Lincoln Hospital
Bronx, New York
Professor of Community and Preventive Medicine
New York Medical College
Valhalla, New York

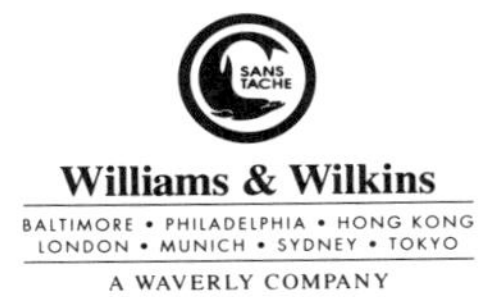

Williams & Wilkins

BALTIMORE • PHILADELPHIA • HONG KONG
LONDON • MUNICH • SYDNEY • TOKYO

A WAVERLY COMPANY

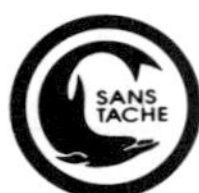

Editor: Tim Satterfield
Associate Editor: Molly L. Mullen
Copy Editor: Candace B. Levy
Illustration Planner: Ray Lowman
Production Coordinator: Kim Nawrozki

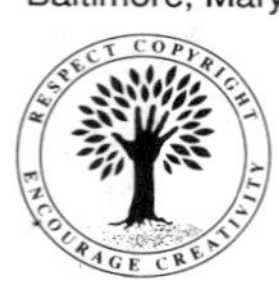

Accurate indications, adverse reactions, and dosage schedules for drugs are provided in this book, but it is possible that they may change. The reader is urged to review the package information data of the manufacturers of the medications mentioned.

Printed in the United States of America

Library of Congress Cataloging in Publication Data

Pousada, Lidia.
Case studies in emergency medicine for the house officer / Lidia Pousada, David B. Levy, Harold H. Osborn.
p. cm. — (Case studies for the house officer series)
Includes index.
Supplement to: Emergency medicine for the house officer / [edited by] Lidia Pousada, Harold H. Osborn, c 1986.
ISBN 0-683-06966-7
1. Emergency medicine—Case studies—Handbooks, manuals, etc. I. Levy, David B. II. Osborn, Harold H. III. Emergency medicine for the house officer. IV. Title. V. Series.
[DNLM: 1. Emergencies—case studies. 2. Emergency Medicine—case studies. WB 105 P878c]
RC86.7.P68 1986 Suppl.
616.02′5—dc20
DNLM/DLC
for Library of Congress 92-48917
CIP

96 97
3 4 5 6 7 8 9 10

Dedicated to

Sara and Anna

Melissa, Jared, and Amanda

Jesse, Kyre, and Kate

Series Editor's Foreword

The series, Case Studies for the House Officer, has been designed to teach medicine by a case study approach. It is considered a supplement to the parent House Officer Series, which provides information in a problem-oriented format. *Emergency Medicine for the House Officer* has proved popular with house officers and medical students. In *Case Studies in Emergency Medicine for the House Officer*, Doctors Pousada, Levy, and Osborn have compiled an impressive series of interesting cases that cover common and uncommon problems seen in the emergency room. They have added thoughtful "Pearls" and "Pitfalls." The book should be a useful and enjoyable learning experience for students of emergency medicine.

Lawrence P. Levitt, M.D.
Senior Consultant in Neurology
Lehigh Valley Hospital Center
Allentown, Pennsylvania

Clinical Professor of Neurology
Hahnemann University and
Clinical Associate Professor
Temple University School of Medicine

About the Authors

Lidia Pousada, MD, FACP is a graduate of the six-year biomedical program at the City College of New York and New York Medical College. Following residency training in internal medicine and primary care at Montefiore Medical Center in the Bronx, she worked for the United States National Health Service Corps in emergency medicine and ambulatory care. Dr. Pousada is board certified in geriatric medicine and until recently occupied the position of Associate Director of the Unified Division of Geriatrics at Montefiore Medical Center/Albert Einstein College of Medicine. She is currently Director of the Division of Geriatrics at New Rochelle Hospital Medical Center in New York and Associate Professor of Medicine at New York Medical College (appointment pending). Her research and teaching interests lie in the field of geriatric emergency medicine.

David Levy, DO is a graduate of Muhlenberg College in Pennsylvania and the University of Osteopathic Medicine and Health Sciences in Des Moines, Iowa. Dr. Levy completed residency training in emergency medicine and served as chief resident in emergency medicine for two years at New York Medical College/Lincoln Hospital. He is currently an Assistant Professor of Emergency Medicine at the Allegheny Campus of the Medical College of Pennsylvania.

Harold H. Osborn, MD, FACEP, FACP, ABMT is an attending physician and Head of Medical Research in the Departments of Emergency Medicine at both Lincoln Hospital and St. Barnabas Hospital, Bronx, New York. He is also Professor of Community and Preventive Medicine at the New York Medical College in Valhalla, New York.

Preface

Recent decades have witnessed an explosion in utilization of emergency services throughout the United States. This trend has coincided with an unprecedented expansion of medical technology to include numerous innovative diagnostic and treatment modalities. During these same years, medicine has been challenged with the appearance of previously unfamiliar syndromes such as acquired immune deficiency. The traditional "Emergency Room" has had to grow into the modern Emergency Department.

As a result, the task of the physician has multiplied exponentially in difficulty. The emergency physician still must excel in the traditional skills of obtaining a medical history and performing a physical examination under exacting time constraints. But in addition, he or she must be fluent with the latest permutations of biomedical technology and their application to the Emergency Department setting.

The cases in this book are for the most part composites of patients seen and treated by the authors. These cases were selected as representative of the depth and breadth of current emergency medicine practice. The authors have attempted to pique the reader's interest, challenge his or her diagnostic skills, and ultimately offer a few words of wisdom culled from years of experience. Although this text cannot substitute for the presence of a seasoned mentor at one's side in the Emergency Department, it is our hope that the exercise of thinking through these cases will supplement that learning process.

Lida Pousada, MD, FACP
David Levy, DO
Harold H. Osborn, MD, FACEP, FACP, ABMT

Acknowledgments

Thanks are due A. J. Smalley, MD, and Nina Gentile, MD, for their additions to the case studies presented in this text.

Most of all, the authors would like to thank the patients of the Bronx as well as the cities of Pittsburgh, Pennsylvania, and Hartford, Connecticut, for their essential contribution of intriguing and instructive case material.

Contents

A FEBRILE INTRAVENOUS DRUG ABUSER

Case 1:

A 24-year-old male presented complaining of fever for the past 24 hours, chills, scant dry cough, and "a very weak feeling." He denied sore throat, stiff neck, ear pain, nasal congestion, shortness of breath, chest pain, dyspnea on exertion, abdominal pain, nausea and vomiting, diarrhea, dysuria or urinary frequency or urgency, weight loss, or rash. He denied any other pertinent medical history. He denied any history of alcohol abuse, but admitted to occasional use of intravenous heroin and cocaine over the past 5 years. His last intravenous injection was 3 days earlier. He had no listed address on his chart and stated that he "stays with friends."

On examination, he was an unkempt and disheveled young man who appeared older than his stated age. He was lying on a stretcher shivering. His blood pressure was 130/70, pulse 96/minute and regular, respiratory rate 12/minute, and rectal temperature 102.2° F. His scleras were anicteric, fundi were benign, tympanic membranes were normal bilaterally, and his pharynx was slightly injected without exudate. His dentition was poor. His neck was supple. Lungs were clear bilaterally. His heart sounds were normal except for a loud P2 and he had a grade I/VI nonradiating systolic ejection murmur along the right sternal border, which increased with inspiration. His abdominal examination was unremarkable. He had no significant lymphadenopathy and no peripheral edema. There were prominent track marks on both arms without any signs of phlebitis or cellulitis. His neurologic examination was entirely unremarkable.

DIAGNOSTIC CLUE:

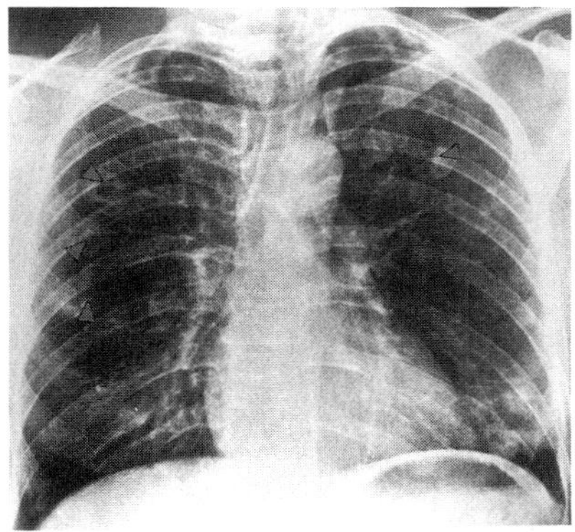

QUESTIONS:

1. What is the likely diagnosis? What is the differential diagnosis of fever in an intravenous drug abuser?

2. What tests should be ordered to work this patient up?

3. If all his test results are normal, does this patient need to be admitted?

4. What are other physical findings that might be associated with the likely diagnosis?

5. What is the appropriate treatment for this patient?

ANSWERS:

1. An intravenous drug abuser with a fever must be presumed to have acute bacterial endocarditis until proven otherwise. This particular patient also has a right-sided murmur, a loud P2, and a chest x-ray consistent with septic emboli to the lungs, findings which further support the diagnosis of drug-related endocarditis. The differential diagnosis covers a broad range of infectious diseases, most notably pneumonia, due to either septic emboli, aspiration, or parasitic infection; meningitis (unlikely in an alert patient without neurologic findings); a cellulitis or septic phlebitis at an injection site; tuberculosis; or hepatitis. In addition, intravenous drug abusers may have underlying AIDS, with all the potential associated infectious diseases, such as Pneumocystis carinii pneumonia, toxoplasmosis, and bacteremia from unknown sources.

2. The patient should have a CBC with differential count and platelets; serum electrolytes, liver function tests, and renal function tests; a sedimentation rate; urinalysis, Gram stain, and urine culture; Gram stain and acid-fast stain of any sputum obtained; and serial blood cultures. If a febrile intravenous drug user has any neurologic symptoms or signs, a CAT scan of the head with contrast should be peformed followed by a lumbar puncture.

3. Even if all the tests ordered are negative, this patient will require admission to rule out bacterial endocarditis as well as other serious infections.

4. Endocarditis may be acute or subacute. Patients with subacute endocarditis frequently have underlying cardiac disease (e.g., rheumatic valvular disease, aortic stenosis, septal defects) and often give a history of recent oropharyngeal surgery, dental procedures, cystoscopy, or bowel instrumentation. The patient's complaints may include low-grade fever, weakness, myalgias, arthralgias, fatigue, and anorexia. Possible physical manifestations include petechiae; subungual splinter hemorrhages; Osler's nodes (painful raised nodules on fingers); Janeway lesions (nontender red papules on palms or soles); retinal hemorrhages and cotton-wool exudates; Roth's spots (retinal white spots surrounded by hemorrhage); septic emboli to the spleen, kidneys, bowel, heart, lungs or brain (with or without subsequent abscess formation); anemia; heart murmurs; glomerulonephritis; and disseminated intravascular coagulation.

In contrast, patients with acute endocarditis generally have an abrupt onset with high fever and shaking chills. Intravenous drug abusers are among those patients who typically present with acute rather than subacute endocarditis. Other than fever, systemic manifestations may be absent and there may be no murmur or a very subtle right-sided murmur.

5. Streptococcus viridans and all other streptococci exclusive of enterococci account for about 40% of all cases of endocarditis. Enterococci are responsible for about 10% of cases. Staphylococcus aureus and epidermidis have become increasingly frequent pathogens, particularly in hospitalized patients and drug abusers, and are the most

common organisms seen with acute endocarditis. Endocarditis due to Gram-negative bacilli such as Pseudomonas species and Serratia marcescens has also increased in frequency in drug-related cases. Other possible Gram-negative bacilli include Neisseria gonorrhoea and Salmonella organisms. Fungal endocarditis may occur in addicts; Candida albicans is seen most often in hospitalized patients, and Candida parapsilosis and other non-albicans species are isolated most frequently from addicts.

Appropriate treatment should include empiric intravenous antibiotic therapy pending results of blood cultures. The empiric antibiotic regimen should include a combination effective against penicillin-sensitive streptococcus, enterococci, and penicillin-resistant staphylococci. One effective regimen would be penicillin G, nafcillin, and gentamicin. Penicillin-allergic patients can be given vancomycin and gentamicin.

PEARLS:

1. Intravenous drug abusers with acute endocarditis generally have right-sided valve involvement with right-sided murmurs. This preferential location is thought to be due to valvular damage by injected particulate matter. Jugular venous distention and giant V waves can be seen in acute tricuspid regurgitation. A loud P2, wide splitting of S2, or a pulmonic flow murmur suggest pulmonary hypertension due to emboli.

2. Always do a rectal temperature before concluding that a patient is not febrile, because oral temperatures (particularly in dyspneic patients) are unreliable.

3. Never discount serious infection because a patient denies recent intravenous drug abuse. The patient may be misrepresenting the facts and still be actively abusing drugs, or may be immunosuppressed and presenting for the first time with a serious infection.

PITFALLS:

1. Patients with endocarditis need not exhibit a murmur upon examination. The murmur may be absent, present, or variable.

2. Signs of right-sided endocarditis are typically difficult to elicit and may be entirely absent. Listen very carefully for murmurs, especially diastolic, and listen for a right-sided S3 or S4.

3. Patients with AIDS can present with bacteremia and sepsis without an obvious source.

REFERENCES:

Hermans PE. The clinical manifestations of infective endocarditis. Mayo Clin Proc 1981;57(1):15-21.

Marantz PR, Linzer M, Feiner CJ, et al. Inability to predict diagnosis in febrile intravenous drug abusers. Ann Int Med 1987;106:823-828.

Panidis IP, Kotler MN, Mintz GS, et al. Right heart endocarditis: clinical and echocardiographic features. Am Heart J 1984;107:759.

Swartz MN. Infective endocarditis. In: Rubinstein E, Federman DD, eds. Medicine. 1987;7(18):1-25.

Wilson WR, Guilani ER, Danielson GK, Geraci JE. General considerations in the diagnosis and treatment of infective endocarditis. Mayo Clin Proc 1982;57(2):81-85.

SORE THROAT AND DYSPNEA

Case 2:

A 29-year-old truck driver presented to the Emergency Department holding his throat and indicating difficulty in breathing and speaking. He had been in good health but awoke that day with a sore throat and general malaise. During the day he experienced increasing difficulty in speaking and breathing and a sensation that his "throat was closing". The patient had a ten pack-year smoking history. He stated he had been treated on one or two occasions in the past for bronchitis but specifically denied a history of asthma or chronic pulmonary disease. He denied any allergies or prior episodes of shortness of breath. He had never been hospitalized and had no other significant illnesses. He stated he had eaten little during the day and had experienced some difficulty swallowing.

On examination, the patient was a muscular, well-nourished individual in mild respiratory distress, breathing rapidly but without stridor. He appeared quite anxious, spoke in muffled tones, and sat upright, leaning forward on the stretcher. His blood pressure was 118/80, pulse 96/minute and regular, respiratory rate 20/minute, and oral temperature 98.3° F. His color was good, his neck was supple, and there was no lymphadenopathy. Examination of the oropharynx revealed erythema without exudate. The tonsils were slightly enlarged. The lung fields were clear bilaterally with good air entry. His heart sounds were normal. The rest of the physical examination was unremarkable. A subsequent rectal temperature was 100.6° F.

Blood chemistries were within normal limits. A CBC revealed a white cell count of 15,000 with 80% polymorphonuclear and 5% band forms. An immediate bedside portable x-ray of the lateral neck was obtained.

DIAGNOSTIC CLUE:

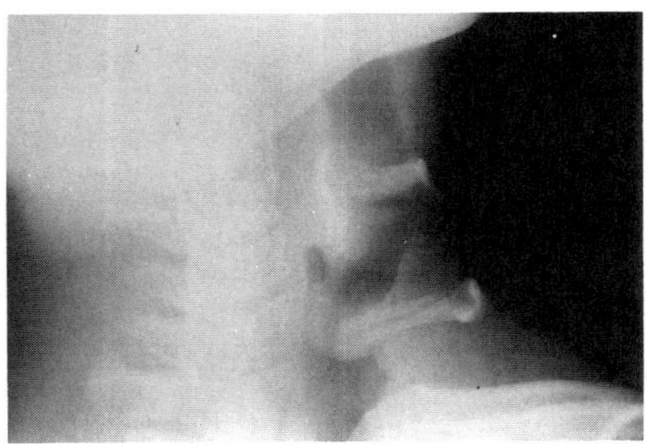

QUESTIONS:

1. What is the correct diagnosis?
2. What is the differential diagnosis of acute airway obstruction?
3. What other diagnostic tests are indicated in the evaluation of this patient?
4. What is the correct approach to airway management in patients with this condition?
5. What additional treatment should be offered this patient?

ANSWERS:

1. The correct diagnosis is acute epiglottitis. The diagnosis is suggested by the history of sore throat and dysphagia and the physical findings of fever and dyspnea in the absence of wheezing. It is confirmed by the x-ray of the lateral neck, which reveals an enlarged, swollen epiglottis. Although epiglottitis has traditionally been considered an illness of children, it occurs in adults and recent reports suggest that its incidence is higher than had been previously suggested. The infection often results in a cellulitis involving all the supraglottic structures, including the arytenoids and aryepiglottic folds and is more correctly termed a supraglottitis. The inflammation and resultant edema in turn create the physical signs and symptoms which (in order of decreasing frequency) are: sore throat, dysphagia, respiratory difficulty, muffled voice, drooling, and stridor. A hoarse voice is atypical and suggests laryngitis or croup. Causative organisms include Haemophilus influenzae, Streptococcus pneumoniae, Haemophilus parainfluenzae, Staphylococcus species, and Neisseria catarrhalis.

2. The differential diagnosis of acute airway obstruction can be divided into infectious and noninfectious causes. From the front of the oropharynx to the back, the infectious possibilities are Ludwig's angina (usually caused by an abscess of the second or third mandibular molar), peritonsillar abscess, diphtheria, lingual tonsillar abscess, retropharyngeal abscess (rare in adults), and laryngotracheitis or croup. The presence of a barking cough and hoarseness suggest the diagnosis of infection of the larynx, while drooling and stridor suggest an infection above the larynx, especially epiglottitis. The noninfectious possibilities include hematoma of the base of the tongue, epiglottic ulcer, vocal cord polyp, foreign body, laryngeal edema (secondary to allergic reactions, smoke inhalation, or thermal injury), hereditary angioneurotic edema, glottic stenosis, trauma to the anterior neck, and asthma or chronic obstructive pulmonary disease.

3. In addition to a complete history, thorough physical examination, and lateral neck film, every patient suspected of having epiglottitis should have direct or indirect laryngoscopy performed. Visualization of the epiglottis is the most reliable way to make the diagnosis and can be easily performed with a fiberoptic laryngoscope. The lateral neck film should be performed first and the examination should take place in the Emergency Department or Operating Room where the patient can be properly observed and a surgical aiway secured if necessary. Positive findings include swelling of the epiglottis, aryepiglottic folds, arytenoids, or uvula and ballooning of the retropharyngeal space. A negative x-ray does not preclude the diagnosis and should be followed by examination of the epiglottis in all suspected cases. Culturing the pharynx or epiglottis has not proved beneficial. Blood cultures, when positive, correlate closely with the causative organism. Bacteremia, especially that due to H. influenzae is associated with a more fulminant course and a high risk of airway obstruction.

4. Patients with suspected epiglottitis should have constant observation and should undergo all tests in the Emergency Department, including x-rays. Although acute airway obstruction has been provoked by examination of the oropharynx in children, there have been no case reports of laryngospasm following examination of an adult. There is an increased margin of safety for physical examination in adults perhaps due to a larger, more rigid upper airway and relatively less reactive lymphoid tissue. Nonetheless, the examination should proceed only after consultation with an ENT specialist and adequate preparation for establishing an emergency artificial airway.

Nasotracheal or endotracheal intubation is the airway of choice. If the patient cannot be intubated, a surgical airway must be secured. Cricothyroidotomy is the preferred surgical airway in the emergency setting. It is technically easier to perform than a tracheostomy and has a lower complication rate. The use of prophylactic airway intervention (early intubation) in all cases of epiglottitis is still controversial. Advocates of the latter approach argue that progression to airway obstruction can occur suddenly and without warning. Aggressive airway management has significantly lowered the mortality among children to less than 1%, and the continued high mortality rate reported in adult series (over 7%) would seem to indicate this approach should be adopted for adults as well.

5. In addition to early intubation and administration of humidified oxygen, patients should be started on intravenous antibiotics after blood cultures are performed. Because of the possibility of beta-lactamase-producing H. influenzae, initial treatment should include ampicillin plus either chloramphenicol or a third-generation cephalosporin active against H. influenzae. Positive culture results can serve as a guide for ongoing therapy. Corticosteroids have been given in the past to patients with respiratory compromise although there is no good evidence that they are efficacious.

PEARLS:

1. The diagnosis of epiglottitis should be suspected in any patient with sore throat and dysphagia whose subjective symptoms are out of proportion to the findings on physical examination of the oropharynx.

2. Airway obstruction and ventilatory compromise, when they occur, usually happen early in the course of epiglottitis. Patients who are not intubated should be closely observed in the Emergency Department or an intensive-care setting. Prophylactic airway protection is the safest approach in managing patients with epiglottitis.

PITFALLS:

1. The absence of respiratory difficulty in no way rules out the diagnosis of epiglottitis. All patients with suspected epiglottitis must have a thorough evaluation, including visualization of the epiglottis.

2. Lateral neck x-rays are positive in 90% of cases when the films are evaluated by experienced personnel. A precise knowledge of local anatomy is essential in evaluating these radiographs. If there is any doubt about the interpretation, the films should be read by an experienced radiologist or an ENT specialist.

3. The diagnosis of epiglottitis should never be excluded on the basis of the x-ray alone. All suspected cases should have laryngoscopic examination.

REFERENCES:

Bromiatowski M. Epiglottitis. Ear Nose Throat J 1985;64(1):22-27.

Mace SE. Acute epiglottitis in adults. Am J Emerg Med 1985;3(6):543-550.

Mayosmith MF, Hirsch PJ, Wodzinski SF, et al. Acute epiglottitis in adults: an eight-year experience in the state of Rhode Island. N Engl J Med 1986;314:1133-1139.

Stankiewicz JA, King Bowes A. Croup and epiglottitis: a radiologic study. Laryngoscope 1985;95(10):1159-1160.

Warner J, Finlay WEI. Fulminating epiglottitis. Anesthesia 1985;40(4):348-352.

CHEST PAIN IN A YOUNG MAN

Case 3:

An anxious 34-year-old male presented complaining of an episode of chest pain 1 hour earlier. He had been mowing the lawn at noon on a hot summer day when he noted the sudden onset of a "heavy feeling" in the middle of his chest. He became slightly short of breath and "broke out into a cold sweat." He sat down, but the pain did not subside; it remained a dull ache for almost 45 minutes before gradually dissipating. He took some Alka-Seltzer without relief.

He had just eaten a large lunch, but denied gastrointestinal discomfort. He denied any previous episodes of chest pain or dyspnea. He stated he was "very athletic" and regularly participated in competitive and endurance sports. He denied any history of hypertension; diabetes; or heart, gastrointestinal or lung disease. No family history was available, as he was adopted. He denied having any friends or family with recent chest pain, although he had been following recent news reports on a major sports figure hospitalized with heart disease. He had never been a smoker, and denied abuse of alcohol or drugs.

On examination, he was a muscular young man in no apparent distress. His blood pressure was 120/84, pulse 58/minute, respiratory rate 12/minute, and oral temperature 98.2° F. His trachea was midline. His lungs were clear bilaterally. His heart sounds were normal, and he had no murmurs, gallops, or rubs. There was no jugular venous distention, hepatomegaly, or peripheral edema. His abdominal exam was unremarkable. His calves were not swollen or tender, and no cords were palpated. Homan's sign was negative bilaterally. Peripheral pulses were normal and bilaterally symmetrical.

DIAGNOSTIC CLUE:

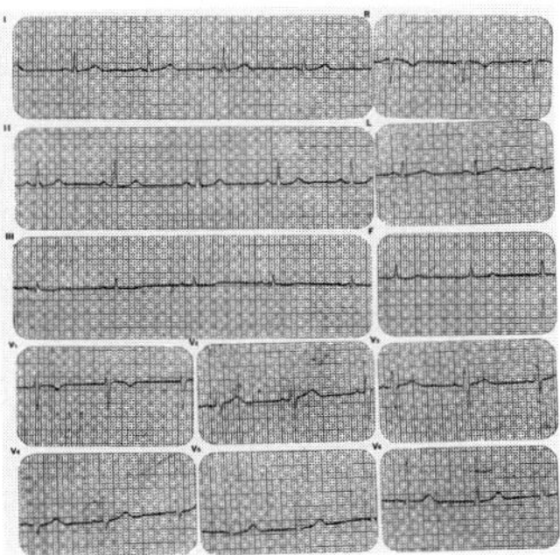

QUESTIONS:

1. What are potentially life-threatening causes of chest pain? What are benign causes of chest pain?

2. What further tests should be ordered to evaluate this patient?

3. If all his test results are normal, does this patient need to be admitted?

4. What is the likely diagnosis in this case?

5. What would be appropriate treatment for this patient?

ANSWERS:

1. When evaluating a patient with chest pain, the main task of the Emergency Department physician is to distinguish between the many minor causes of chest pain and the few potentially serious conditions. The following potentially life-threatening disorders must be ruled out before the patient's symptoms can be ascribed to a benign etiology.

a. Unstable angina (includes new onset and crescendo)
b. Myocardial infarction
c. Dissecting aortic aneurysm
d. Pneumothorax
e. Pulmonary embolus
f. Pericarditis
g. Pneumonia

An easy method for remembering benign causes of chest pain is to start at the skin and work through layer by layer to the back. The following are the most common causes:

a. Musculoskeletal strain
b. Calcific tendonitis
c. Cervical and thoracic nerve root pain
d. Costochondritis
e. Thoracic outlet syndrome
f. Rib fractures
g. Gastrointestinal problems (reflux esophagitis, gastritis, ulcer, gallbladder disease, pancreatitis)
h. Tracheobronchitis
i. Pleurisy
j. Stable angina

2. It would be prudent to order a chest x-ray and a blood gas. An abnormally low pO_2 would dictate the need for a lung scan. Cardiac enzymes with MB fractionation could be sent as baseline studies. If the patient remained in the Emergency Department for any length of time, the enzymes would need to be repeated serially. Serial CPK-MB sampling using immunochemical assays has recently been shown to be useful in the diagnosis of myocardial infarction in patients with nondiagnostic EKGs.

3. Patients in whom myocardial ischemia is a primary diagnostic consideration should be admitted on the basis of the history alone. It is entirely possible to have acute myocardial ischemia with a normal EKG. The accuracy of diagnosis of acute myocardial infarction by electrocardiography is no greater than 80%. Other patients with myocardial ischemic pain who should be admitted include new onset angina (less than 2 weeks' duration), unstable angina (increase in duration, frequency, or severity of stable angina), angina unrelieved by nitroglycerin, or angina lasting more than 30 minutes.

4. Although this patient is young for heart disease, his history is a classic description of an acute myocardial infarction. Since we have no family history, it is possible that other members of his natural family suffered premature atherosclerosis and cardiac ischemia and that he is at risk for early myocardial infarction. His electrocardiogram is normal, but acute ischemia has not been ruled out. Another diagnostic possibility is pulmonary embolus. However, he has no obvious source (such as a thrombophlebitis) and he is neither tachypneic nor tachycardic on examination, making pulmonary embolus a less likely possibility. Spontaneous pneumothorax is seen more commonly in males and is most often due to spontaneous rupture of subpleural blebs. His breath sounds are not decreased, nor is he tachypneic on exam, but a chest x-ray should be done to rule out a small pneumothorax. He has no fever or signs of infection on examination. He has no signs of local trauma or tenderness. There is no obvious gastrointestinal source.

5. Assuming that all the patient's tests are normal, he will require observation to rule out acute myocardial infarction. Some Emergency Departments have the capacity to keep patients for observation for 12 to 24 hours. In that event, he should be placed on a cardiac monitor and observed, with repeat cardiac isoenzymes and electrocardiograms at specified intervals. If the Emergency Department does not have that capacity, the patient should be admitted to a monitored bed for serial enzymes and electrocardiograms. At present, the patient is in no pain and requires no other medical intervention.

PEARLS:

1. In an acute myocardial infarction, the MB fraction may rise before the total CPK value, and total CPK and MB fraction may not be elevated early in the course of an infarction.

2. It is prudent to admit all patients with new onset angina of less than 2 weeks' duration.

3. Always ask about hidden risk factors such as drug use and especially cocaine use, since cocaine can precipitate myocardial infarction in an otherwise healthy individual.

PITFALLS:

1. Do not assume that patients with equivocal histories are unlikely to have myocardial ischemia. These patients often require admission for observation precisely because their histories are equivocal.

2. Chest pain in pneumothorax need not be pleuritic; it may be described as a "crushing" pain or a severe dull ache.

3. A patient with a history consistent with myocardial ischemia should not have that history discounted on the basis of anterior chest wall tenderness. Costochondritis is

greatly overdiagnosed in the absence of the local warmth, erythema, swelling and tenderness originally described by Tietze.

4. Beware of chest pain radiating to the back, as this may signal an aortic dissection. When evaluating a patient with this complaint, the physician should be sure to obtain blood pressures in both arms, compare pulses in all extremities, and check a CXR for signs of dissection.

REFERENCES:

Braunwald E. The aggressive treatment of acute myocardial infarction. Circulation 1985;71:1087.

Brush JE Jr, Brand DA, Acampora D, et al. Use of the initial electrocardiogram to predict in-hospital complications of acute myocardial infarction. N Engl J Med 1985;312:1137.

Fisher ML, Keleman MH, Collins D, et al. Routine serum enzyme tests in the diagnosis of acute myocardial infarction: cost-effectiveness. Arch Intern Med 1983;143:1541.

Hurst JW, King SB III, Friesinger GC, et al. Atherosclerotic coronary heart disease: recognition, prognosis, and treatment. In: Hurst JW, Logue RB, Rackley CB, et al, eds. The Heart 6th ed. New York: McGraw-Hill, 1986.

Roberts R. The two out of three criteria for the diagnosis of infarction: is it passe? Chest 1984;86:511.

Siber WB, Lewis LM, Erb RE, et al. Early detection of acute myocardial infarction in patients presenting with chest pain and non-diagnostic ECGs. Ann Emerg Med 1990;19:1359.

Sibler WB, Lewis LM, Erb RE, et al. Early detection of acute myocardial infarction in patients presenting with chest pain and non-diagnostic ECGs. Ann Emerg Med 19: 1359, 1990.

CARDIAC ARREST

Case 4:

A 52-year-old male presented to the Emergency Department complaining of nausea and lightheadedness of 2 hours' duration. These symptoms began after the patient awoke at approximately 6:00 am. He had a history of a myocardial infarction 3 years earlier, and was currently taking verapamil three times a day and nitroglycerin as needed. He stated that he felt well the previous day and had not required any nitroglycerin for 2 weeks.

On physical examination, he was a mildly obese male who appeared anxious. Vital signs were pulse 150/minute and regular, blood pressure 98/74, and respirations 20/minute and not labored. His skin was cool and dry, there was minimal neck vein distention, and the lungs were clear except for some bibasilar crackles. The heart was tachycardic but regular, with a variable first heart sound and no murmurs or extra heart sounds. There was no lower extremity edema or cyanosis.

An electrocardiogram from 1 year ago was reported to show normal sinus rhythm with first-degree heart block, a QRS interval of 0.10 second, a normal axis, and Q waves present in leads V_1 to V_4.

Fifteen minutes after the patient's arrival, he became unresponsive and pulseless.

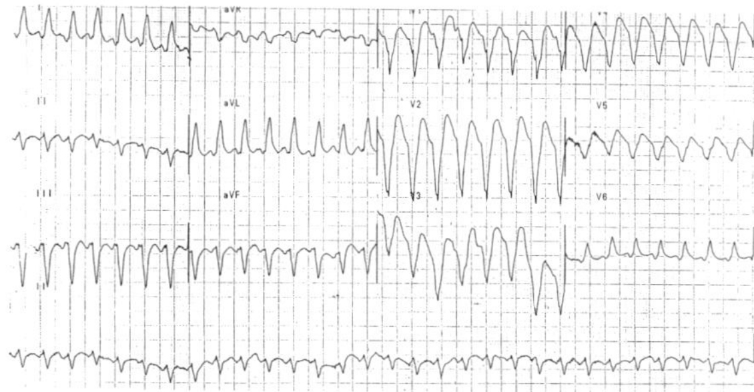

DIAGNOSTIC CLUES:

1. EKG taken initially in ED

2. Rhythm strip taken when the patient became unresponsive

QUESTIONS:

1. What is the correct interpretation of the initial electrocardiogram?

2. What treatment is indicated?

3. What rhythm is seen on the second electrocardiogram?

4. What should be the initial treatment of the second rhythm?

5. What role is there for administration of epinephrine and sodium bicarbonate in cardiac arrest?

ANSWERS:

1. The patient is in a wide QRS complex tachycardia. The differential diagnosis is ventricular tachycardia versus a supraventricular tachycardia with aberrant conduction due to either a bundle branch block or accessory pathway. It is important to distinguish between these two because inappropriate treatment can cause a rapid deterioration in the patient's condition, resulting in cardiac arrest.

In order to distinguish if the rhythm is supraventricular or ventricular in origin, the physician must approach the patient in a systematic manner. Physical examination should establish the presence or absence of cannon "a" waves in the neck veins and should include auscultation for variation of the first heart sound. Either of these findings indicates dissociation between the atria and ventricles, suggesting ventricular tachycardia. Electrocardiogram factors favoring ventricular tachycardia are concordant positivity or concordant negativity in the precordial leads, QRS complex with a left axis, QRS interval greater than 0.14 seconds, fusion beats, and evidence of independent atrial activity.

The QRS morphology also provides important clues. The diagnosis of ventricular tachycardia is favored if the QRS complex in V_1 is a single peak or has an RSR′ complex where the R complex is of greater amplitude than R′. A RSR′ configuration in V_1 where R′ is of greater amplitude than R favors aberrant conduction. In V_6, an rS or a QS complex usually indicates ventricular ectopy. A triphasic (qRs) complex in V_6 suggests supraventricular tachycardia with aberrant conduction.

In this patient, the width of the complexes (greater than 0.14 seconds) and the morphology of the complexes in V_1 and V_6 make ventricular tachycardia the most likely diagnosis.

2. The most important determinant of treatment in a patient with a wide complex tachycardia is the clinical status of the patient. If the patient is determined to be unstable because of persistent symptoms (chest pain, dyspnea); hypotension (systolic blood pressure less than 90 mm Hg); or the presence of congestive heart failure, ischemia or infarction, then electrical cardioversion is indicated. Unless it is contraindicated, intravenous sedation should be administered to the conscious patient before cardioversion. Diazepam and midazolam are useful agents in this setting. Vital signs must be closely monitored. The patient should already be on a cardiac monitor with supplemental oxygen and intravenous access established and ventilatory support readily available. It is possible for a patient to degenerate into ventricular fibrillation after attempted cardioversion.

For the patient who is determined to be clinically stable, chemical cardioversion can be attempted with lidocaine or procainamide. Lidocaine is traditionally used as the first-line agent and administered as a 1 mg/kg intravenous bolus. If there is no response, lidocaine is repeated as a 0.5 mg/kg bolus every 5 to 10 minutes to a maximum of 3 mg/kg.

If there is no response to lidocaine, procainamide can be administered. Many clinicians elect to administer procainamide as a first-line agent for wide QRS complex tachycardias when the etiology is uncertain since it is effective for both atrial and ventricular arrhythmias, as well as supraventricular tachycardia with an accessory pathway.

For the patient in this case, a brief attempt with an antiarrhythmic may be warranted, but the clinician should be ready to proceed quickly to cardioversion (usually starting at 50 joules), since patients with ventricular tachycardia and ischemic heart disease have a high mortality if not treated aggressively.

3. This rhythm is ventricular fibrillation, the most common cause of primary cardiac arrest Ventricular fibrillation is a life-threatening emergency since there is no organized pattern of contraction of myocardial cells and thus no forward blood flow. However, it is the most salvageable rhythm of cardiac arrest if rapid treatment is initiated.

4. Among all the current recommended therapies, early defibrillation is the single most important intervention for resuscitation of patients from cardiac arrest. Defibrillation must take precedence in the management of ventricular fibrillation and should be implemented before institution of CPR, insertion of intravenous lines, delivery of drugs, or endotracheal intubation. As proven in prehospital and hospital cardiac arrest experience, the success of resuscitation of patients with ventricular fibrillation is determined by the speed with which electrical defibrillation is initiated. The longer ventricular fibrillation is allowed to persist, the greater the degree of myocardial deterioration and the smaller the likelihood that defibrillation will be successful.

Current ACLS standards recommend initial defibrillation at 200 joules, and if no response, a second defibrillation attempt at 200 to 300 joules, followed by a third attempt at 360 joules if there is still no response.

5. Epinephrine has been administered in the setting of cardiopulmonary resuscitation for years. Only recently have its effects been understood. We now recognize that the main benefit of epinephrine is through its alpha effects, causing peripheral vasoconstriction, which improves coronary and cerebral perfusion pressures. The coronary perfusion pressure is the difference between the aortic diastolic pressure and right atrial diastolic pressure. It is this value which is the most critical predictor of the return of spontaneous circulation. Recent studies have indicated that the current ACLS recommended doses of epinephrine (0.5 to 1.0 mg) are suboptimal and that dosages up to 200 μg/kg (15 mg for a 70 kg patient) are required to obtain optimal blood flow through the heart. More studies

are required to determine if this increase in epinephrine dosage will improve neurologically intact survival.

The liberal use of sodium bicarbonate has been deemphasized. Most resuscitation researchers question whether there is any role for sodium bicarbonate in the uncomplicated cardiac arrest patient. Initial acidemia in the setting of cardiac arrest is usually respiratory, with metabolic acidosis secondary to inadequate perfusion occurring later. While sodium bicarbonate will buffer metabolic acidosis by reacting with hydrogen ions to form water and carbon dioxide, it is the production of carbon dioxide that has been demonstrated to be harmful. The carbon dioxide generated diffuses rapidly into myocardial cells resulting in myocardial dysfunction. Sodium bicarbonate also results in hyperosmolality, which is a negative predictor of survival. Finally, while acidosis may blunt catecholamine response (an effect which is overcome by administration of higher doses of epinephrine), it also has beneficial effects (e.g., improved oxygen delivery to tissues and possible myocardial protective effects). Acidemia in the setting of cardiac arrest is best treated by improving ventilation and restoring circulation.

PEARLS:

1. The most crucial determinant of outcome following cardiac arrest is the interval of time from collapse to the provision of definitive care.

2. Ventricular fibrillation accounts for up to two-thirds of prehospital witnessed arrests.

3. In a study of 200 patients with wide complex tachycardia, the odds were approximately 5:1 in favor of ventricular tachycardia.

4. Always ask the patient with wide complex tachycardia two questions: Is there a history of previous myocardial infarction? Was that infarction followed by a rapid heartbeat? If the answer to both is yes, it is almost certain that the current episode is ventricular tachycardia.

PITFALLS:

1. Do not be fooled by an alert, asymptomatic patient. Ventricular tachycardia can be well tolerated.

2. Do not administer verapamil to a patient with a wide QRS complex tachycardia without definite evidence of supraventricular tachycardia with aberrancy. Because definite evidence of aberrancy is often impossible, many authorities now feel that adenosine is

a more appropriate agent. Verapamil also should not be given to a patient with supraventricular tachycardia and a history of preexcitation syndrome, as it may precipitate ventricular tachycardia.

3. Never initiate treatment for a presumed arrhythmia before confirming vital signs and ruling out the possibility of electrocardiogram artifact.

4. Avoid administration of sodium bicarbonate early in cardiac arrest.

5. Do not forget to adjust lidocaine dosage for the elderly patient or the patient with congestive heart failure or liver disease.

REFERENCES:

Callahan ML. High dose epinephrine therapy and other advances in treating cardiac armrest. West J Med 1990;152:697-703.

Guerci AD, Chardia N, Johnson E, et al. Failure of sodium bicarbonate to improve resuscitation from ventricular fibrillation in dogs. Circulation 1986;74(4):75-79.

Ottis CW, Yakaitas RW. The role of epinephrine in CPR: a reappraisal. Ann Intern Med 1984:13:840-843.

Paradis NA, Martin GB, Rivers EP, et al. Coronary perfusion pressure and the return of spontaneous circulation in human cardiopulmonary resuscitation. JAMA 1990;263:1106-1113.

Standards and guidelines for cardiopulmonary resuscitation (CPR) and emergency cardiac care (ECC). JAMA 1986;255:2841-3044.

Wellens H, Bar F, Lie K: The value of the electrocardiogram in the differential diagnosis of a tachycardia with a widened QRS complex. Am J Med 1978; 64:27-33.

A MAN WITH ACUTE ABDOMINAL PAIN

Case 5:

A 41-year-old male presented with abdominal pain of 6 hours' duration. He was in his usual state of good health when he awoke from sleep with epigastric pain of sudden onset, which he described as "stabbing," "very severe," and radiating to his back. He vomited shortly afterwards, and the vomitus contained digested food without blood, "coffee grounds," or bile. The pain was unrelieved, and his wife called an ambulance. By the time he arrived in the Emergency Department, the pain had spread into his chest and he had begun to feel dizzy. His past medical history was remarkable only for hypertension, moderately well-controlled for the past 10 years. He had no family history of cardiac disease. He denied any history of alcohol use; however, he stated he had used intravenous drugs for 2 years, 20 years previously. He had completed a drug rehabilitation program at that time, obtained a college degree, and worked as a computer programmer for the past 10 years. His only medication was propranolol 80 mg bid.

On examination, he was a well-developed black male who appeared in severe pain, lying very quietly on a stretcher. His blood pressure was 170/100, his pulse was 110/minute and regular, his respiratory rate was 20/minute, and he was afebrile. His scleras were anicteric and fundi remarkable only for mild arteriovenous nicking. His neck was supple without adenopathy or tracheal deviation. His lungs were clear bilaterally. His heart sounds were normal, with a grade II/VI systolic ejection murmur at the base and a grade I/IV high-pitched diastolic murmur at the left lower sternal border. There was no gallop, rub, or thrill. His abdomen was soft, with mild epigastric tenderness on palpation and normal bowel sounds. There was no hepatosplenomegaly or mass. Rectal exam revealed brown, heme-negative stool. His extremities were not cyanotic or edematous. Neurologic examination was unremarkable.

An electrocardiogram showed sinus tachycardia with normal intervals and axis. Bloods were drawn, an intravenous line was started, and the patient was sent for x-rays. Shortly after the x-rays were completed, the patient suddenly became hypotensive, with a systolic blood pressure of 80.

DIAGNOSTIC CLUES:

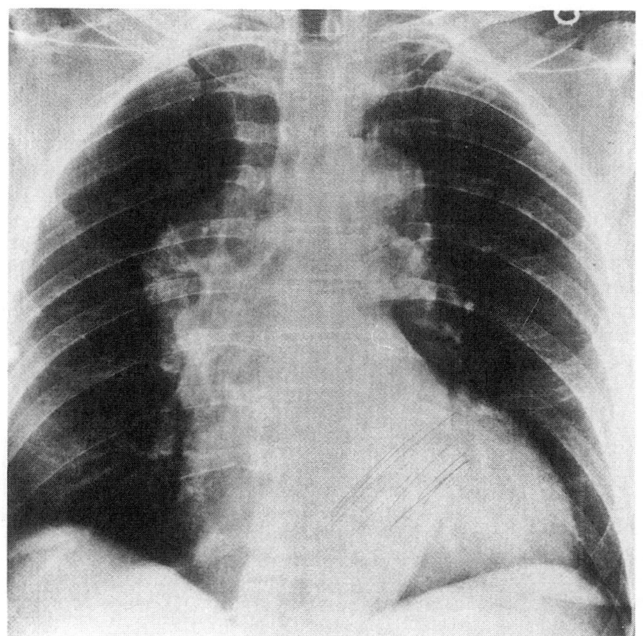

QUESTIONS:

1. What is the diagnosis?
2. What risk factors for this diagnosis does this patient have?
3. What further corroborative tests need to be obtained?
4. What other physical findings might be associated with this diagnosis?
5. What is the appropriate treatment for this patient?

ANSWERS:

1. His abdominal film is unremarkable, but his chest x-ray shows a widened mediastinum. Given the acute onset of chest and epigastric pain along with a murmur of aortic regurgitation and hypotension, the diagnosis must be acute aortic dissection. Although aortic dissection can be silent, over 90% of patients report acute severe chest pain which is "tearing" or "ripping" in quality and usually in the precordial or interscapular areas. Aortic dissection may mimic acute myocardial infarction, pulmonary embolus, esophagitis, peptic ulcer disease, acute cholecystitis, pancreatitis, or renal colic. In cases where the diagnosis is unclear, the rapid onset of pain as well as its severity and location should increase the index of suspicion for acute dissection.

2. Although aortic dissection is not common, at least 10 to 20 cases present yearly to major hospital Emergency Departments. Men are affected in over 65% of cases, and most cases occur in patients aged 40 to 60. Acute aortic dissection can be seen in association with such conditions as Marfan's syndrome, bicuspid aortic valve, Turner's syndrome, and pregnancy. Atherosclerosis is not considered a predisposing factor. Systemic hypertension is the most common finding in patients with acute aortic dissection.

3. Most typically, patients will present with acute severe chest pain, hypertension, a normal EKG, and a widened mediastinum on chest x-ray. Physical examination is often unhelpful, but may reveal asymmetric or absent pulses, asymmetric blood pressure in the upper extremities, or a new murmur of aortic regurgitation. The gold standard for diagnosis remains contrast aortography. Contrast CAT scan can be used as a rapid screening test when the diagnosis is unclear, but an aortogram may still be needed if the anatomy is not defined well. Echocardiography at this time is neither sensitive nor specific enough for diagnostic use. MRI scans are too time-consuming to be of value.

4. Other physical findings associated with acute aortic dissection depend on the site of dissection. Dissection involving the aortic root may lead to acute aortic regurgitation or acute congestive heart failure. Involvement of the carotid or innominate arteries results in decreased level of consciousness or hemiplegia. Disruption of subclavian or iliac arteries may cause acute upper or lower extremity ischemia. Acute intestinal ischemia occurs if the visceral arteries are involved. Anuria, hematuria, and/or flank pain can be seen with renal artery compromise. Less commonly, aortic dissection may cause arrhythmias or myocardial ischemia from coronary artery involvement, superior venal caval syndrome due to compression, dyspnea due to tracheal or bronchial compression, vocal cord paralysis from stretching of the recurrent laryngeal nerve, or Horner's syndrome from compression of the superior cervical ganglion.

5. Acute aortic dissection is a true medical emergency. Patients with dissections involving the ascending aorta usually require immediate surgical repair following medical tabilization. All patients will need maximal monitoring in an intensive-care setting, generally with Swan-Ganz catheterization and arterial lines. The mainstay of therapy

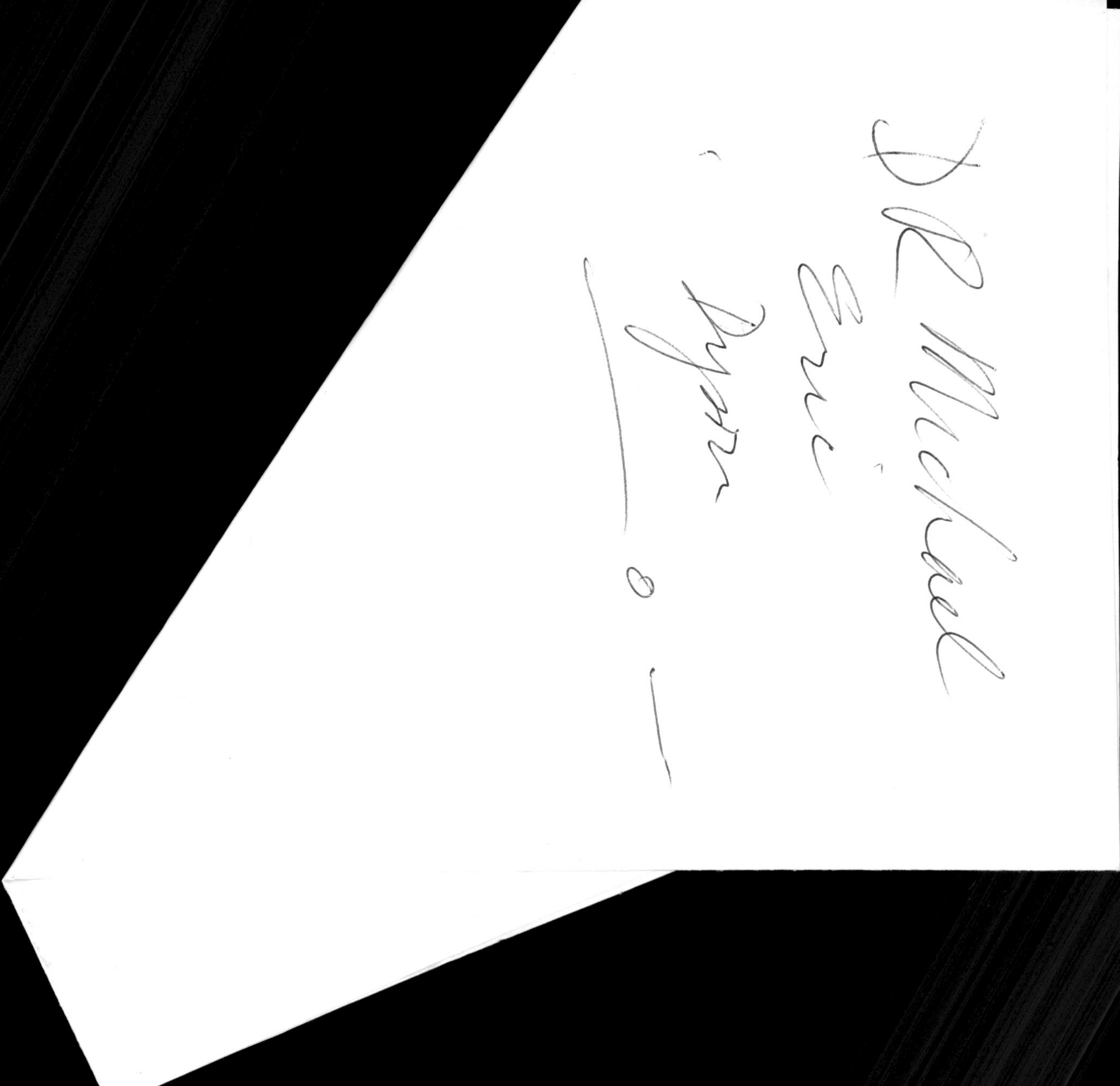

List O' Stuff

- VR Headset
- Vape mod
- Dolls kill clot
- Coke

consists of controlling systemic blood pressure in order to prevent extension of the dissection and possibly avoid rupture. Therapy can be started with IV nitroprusside at 1 to 3 μg/kg/min. Trimethaphan, a ganglionic blocker, may well be the drug of choice fo dissection since it will reduce blood pressure and prevent reflex changes in wall tension. It can be administered intravenously at 0.2 to 6.0 μg/min.

Concomitant beta blockade is essential to decrease peak aortic dP/dt and decrease shearing forces. Propranolol is given in IV increments of 0.5 to 1.0 mg every 2 to 5 minutes until the mean arterial pressure is 60 to 70 mm Hg, the heart rate is less than 60, or other side effects supervene; it is then continued at 2 to 5 mg IV every 1 to 2 hours as needed. Labetolol, which combines alpha and beta blockade, may be preferable, although its half-life is longer than that of propranolol and titration is less precise. An initial dose of 20 mg IV is followed by 20 to 40 mg every 5 to 10 minutes until blood pressure is stabilized, and then every 4 hours as needed. Alternatively, labetolol can be infused intravenously at a rate of 2 to 3 mg/min.

PEARLS:

1. Type A (proximal) dissections are those which involve the ascending aorta; type B (distal) dissections do not.

2. Type A dissections are often rapidly fatal and require surgical intervention. Type B dissections are best managed medically. In either case, a cardiothoracic surgeon should be consulted as soon as the diagnosis is entertained.

3. Initial management is the same for all aortic dissections.

PITFALLS:

1. A normal chest x-ray does not rule out acute aortic dissection.

2. Nitroprusside should not be used without beta blockade because its arteriolar vasodilator effects will increase aortic dP/dt and increase shearing force.

3. Surgical repair palliates but does not "cure" aortic dissection; these patients need close medical follow-up indefinitely.

REFERENCES:

Acute aortic dissection. Lancet 1988;2(8615):827-828.

Crawford ES. The diagnosis and management of aortic dissection. JAMA 1990; 264(19): 2537-2541.

Doroghazi RM, Slater EE, DeSanctis RW, et al. Long-term survival of patients with treated aortic dissection. J Am Coll Cardiol 1984;3:1026-1034.

Graham D, Alexander JJ, Franceschi D, Rashad F. The management of localized abdominal aortic dissections. J Vasc Surg 1988;8(5):582-591.

Moreno-Cabral CE, Miller DC. Diagnosis and management of acute aortic dissections. Choices Cardiol 1989;3(2):66-70.

LETHARGY AND CONFUSION

Case 6:

A 45-year-old woman was brought to the Emergency Department by her son, who noted that she had become increasingly lethargic and confused over the past month to the point where he had been unable to converse logically with her that morning. He stated she had enjoyed excellent health for many years. Approximately 1 month earlier, she began to complain of constant fatigue and vague aches which he attributed to "getting older." Two weeks earlier, she commented that she was suffering from constipation and was not obtaining relief from over-the-counter remedies. One week ago, she "came down with the flu" and went to bed complaining of diffuse aches, weakness, and chills. She stayed in bed, becoming progressively more lethargic, until her son found her unable to hold a conversation with him that morning and brought her to the hospital for evaluation. Her past medical history was notable only for a hysterectomy 3 years earlier. She was born in North Carolina, had two sons, and worked full-time as a kindergarten teacher.

On examination, she was a thin black woman lying quietly on a stretcher. Her blood pressure was 130/70, her pulse was 90/minute and regular, her respiratory rate was 16/minute, and she was afebrile. Her hair was thin, but there were no patches of alopecia. Her extraocular movements were intact, her scleras were anicteric, and her fundi were benign. Her parotid glands were not enlarged and her pharynx was not erythematous. Her neck was supple, with no thyromegaly.

Her lungs were clear bilaterally, and her heart sounds were normal without murmur or gallop. Her abdomen was soft and nontender, with normal bowel sounds. There was no hepatosplenomegaly or mass. Her rectal exam was notable for hard, brown, heme-negative stool. Her extremities were not edematous. She had no significant adenopathy. Neurologic examination was difficult because the patient could not cooperate. She appeared to have diffusely diminished muscle strength and normal response to pinprick throughout. Her deep tendon reflexes were barely elicitable. Cerebellar function and gait could not be tested. She was oriented only to self and could not answer simple questions appropriately.

DIAGNOSTIC CLUES:

Sodium: 148
Chloride: 108
Potassium: 4.8
Bicarbonate: 27
BUN: 24
Creatinine: 1.4
Calcium: 14.5

QUESTIONS:

1. What is the differential diagnosis of this patient's problem?

2. What further tests need to be done?

3. What are other signs and symptoms this patient might exhibit?

4. What is the appropriate immediate treatment for this patient?

ANSWERS:

1. Hypercalcemia can be due to increased intestinal absorption of calcium, increased mobilization of body calcium stores (primarily bone), and decreased renal calcium excretion. Causes of increased intestinal absorption include milk-alkali syndrome (abnormally high dietary calcium intake), vitamin D intoxication, and sarcoidosis (increased sensitivity of the intestine to vitamin D). Bony release of calcium occurs with tumors metastatic to bone, multiple myeloma, lymphoma (due to osteoclast activating factor), hyperthyroidism, primary and secondary hyperparathyroidism, ectopic hyper-parathyroidism secondary to tumor, immobilization, and Paget's disease. Decreased renal excretion of calcium occurs in benign familial hypocalciuric hypercalcemia and with the use of thiazide diuretics. Sarcoid occurs most often in blacks and has a particularly high incidence in North Carolina.

2. The patient needs a chest x-ray and a KUB, looking for hilar adenopathy, lung lesions, kidney stones, nephrocalcinosis, and pancreatic and other soft tissue calcifications. In addition, skull and thoracolumbar spine films can show Paget's disease, multiple myeloma, osteoporosis, and tumor metastases. Hand x-rays will reveal the subperiosteal resorption characteristic of hyperparathyroidism. Additional blood tests to be obtained include serum alkaline phosphatase, albumin, phosphorus, and protein as well as a CBC and a sedimentation rate. If no source is found, additional tests which will need to be done include thyroid function tests, serum PTH, and a 24-hour urine calcium.

3. Signs and symptoms of hypercalcemia include polyuria, polydipsia, nausea, vomiting, abdominal pain, constipation, decreased muscle tone and strength, fatigue, depression, decreased appetite and weight loss. Patients may become lethargic, confused, hallucinatory, obtunded, or comatose. Physical signs include decreased alertness, decreased muscle strength, and depressed reflexes. EKG abnormalities include QT interval shortening, ST segment coving, and T wave widening.

4. Treatment of hypercalcemia begins with intravenous normal saline at a rate of 150 to 250 cc/hour. The normal saline causes calciuresis in an exchange of sodium for calcium. Furosemide 40 to 100 mg as an intravenous bolus (or other loop diuretics) can be added to prevent development of fluid overload and to further increase natriuresis and calciuresis. Serum calcium and fluid balance should be monitored closely.

Specific therapies can be initiated once the source of the hypercalcemia is identified. Steroids are effective in treating the hypercalcemia of sarcoidosis, hypervitaminoses A and D, multiple myeloma, leukemia, and breast cancer. The mechanism of action is inhibition of bone resorption and of gastrointestinal absorption of calcium. The dose of hydocortisone is 25 to 100 mg intravenously every 6 to 8 hours.

Chemotherapeutic agents such as mithramycin can be used to definitively control otherwise resistant tumor hypercalcemia by decreasing bone resorption. Daily doses of 15 to 25 µg/kg administered intravenously over 3 hours are effective. Calcitonin, also an osteoclast inhibitor, is less toxic than mithramycin and may be used for tumor hypercalcemia in doses of 0.5 to 4 MRC units/kg intramuscularly every twelve hours.

Nonsteroidal antiinflammatory agents can be effective in counteracting prostaglandin-mediated tumor hypercalcemia (e.g., breast neoplasms). Indomethacin 25 mg can be given orally in patients without peptic ulcer disease or gastrointestinal bleeding. Intravenous phosphates and EDTA or oral phosphosoda can be used because of the possibility of a rapid fall in serum calcium and tissue deposition of calcium phosphate.

PEARLS:

1. The hypercalcemia of hyperparathyroidism is often associated with a decreased serum phosphate, due to the tendency of parathyroid hormone to decrease tubular reabsorption of phosphate.

2. Remember that rehydration is the most important therapeutic measure for hypercalcemia, regardless of the cause.

3. If the patient is hypoalbuminemic, total calcium levels may be normal despite an elevated ionized calcium level.

PITFALLS:

1. Do not allow the product of the serum calcium and phosphate to exceed 50, as the likelihood of metastatic calcification exists at an elevated calcium-phosphate product.

2. Watch fluid status closely. Patients with marginal cardiac reserve or renal failure can rapidly become fluid overloaded and develop frank congestive heart failure.

REFERENCES:

Muggia FM. Overview of cancer-related hypercalcemia: epidemiology and etiology. Semin Oncol 1990;17(2 suppl 5):3-9.

Pont A. Unusual causes of hypercalcemia. Endocrinol Metab Clin North Am 1989;18(3):753-764.

Ralston SH, Gallacher SJ, Patel U, et al. Cancer-associated hypercalcemia: mobidity and mortality. Clinical experience in 126 treated patients. Ann Intern Med 1990;112(7):499-504.

A PARANOID MIDDLE-AGED WOMAN

Case 7:

A 62-year-old Hispanic female was brought into the Emergency Department by her two daughters, who stated their mother had become increasingly agitated and paranoid over the previous 2 to 3 months. She had been in her usual state of good health until 3 months earlier, when her family noted that she seemed "nervous." She had always been energetic, but she now became very preoccupied with cleanliness, doing and redoing housekeeping chores. She became extremely active in church activities, to the point where she was heavily overcommitted. Her daughters noted she began to neglect her personal appearance and appeared to have lost some weight. Approximately 2 weeks earlier, she began to talk constantly, even when no one was with her. That day, one of her daughters found her speaking somewhat incoherently, crying out that some people were after her and trying to kill her. She had no past medical or psychiatric history and was taking no medications.

On physical examination, she was a thin, agitated woman who appeared frightened. Her blood pressure was 150/100, her pulse was 120 and regular, her respiratory rate was 20/minute, and her temperature was 99° F. Her hair was thick and full, but disheveled. She had slight bilateral exophthalmos without lidlag. Her neck was supple without adenopathy, and her thyroid was not enlarged upon palpation. Her lungs were clear, her heart sounds were normal, and the abdominal exam was unremarkable. Her extremities were notable for a moderate amount of nonpitting edema bilaterally. On neurological exam, her mental status appeared normal, although assessment was difficult because she was very anxious, her speech was pressured and she kept slipping into Spanish. Her sensory and motor exam were normal. Her gait was unremarkable, and cerebellar function appeared intact. Her deep tendon reflexes were diffusely hyperactive without clonus. She had a moderately fine resting tremor in her hands.

DIAGNOSTIC CLUE:

Chest x-ray:

Slightly rotated film with good penetration; soft tissue and bone unremarkable; lung fields clear, without evidence of acute infiltrate; mediastinal mass consistent with substernal goiter; heart size upper limits of normal.

QUESTIONS:

1. What are possible causes of this woman's paranoia?
2. What further tests should be ordered?
3. Which consultants' opinions might be of use?
4. What is the appropriate treatment?
5. What other physical findings might be associated with the likely diagnosis?

ANSWERS:

1. Possible causes of paranoid ideation include paranoid schizophrenia, paranoid personality disorder, dementia with paranoid ideation, and organic causes of paranoid ideation, most notably hyperthyroidism. Late-onset schizophrenia can occur in the elderly, but is characterized by a thought disturbance, which is not described in this patient. A paranoid personality is generally present throughout life and does not usually begin in the later decades.

Dementia often presents not only with memory loss but also with paranoid ideation and even frank hallucinations, usually visual in nature. However, cognitive loss is the sine qua non for the diagnosis of dementia. This patient has not demonstrated any decline in cognitive function either by history or on examination; however, the language barrier may have obscured the exam.

Hyperthyroidism is well-known as a cause of anxiety and even frank psychosis. This patient's physical examination is highly suggestive of hyperthyroidism: she has weight loss, tachycardia, bilateral exophthalmos, hyperreflexia, a fine resting tremor, and pretibial myxedema. Although she does not have an enlarged thyroid on examination, her chest film reveals a substernal goiter.

2. Serum T_4 (thyroxine) and TSH (thyroid stimulating hormone) levels need to be drawn in this patient. However, it is important to remember that serum T_4 may be markedly elevated in postmenopausal women in the absence of hyperthyroidism; the mechanism of this elevation is unclear. Typically, serum TSH levels are normal in these patients. In addition, it has been reported that a large percentage of patients with acute psychiatric disease present with elevations of T_4, probably as a response to stress. These patients will have a normal TSH, whereas patients with true hyperthyroidism will have an elevated T_4 and a suppressed TSH.

A ^{131}I uptake is an important test in the diagnosis of hyperthyroidism. This test will not only definitively identify a substernal goiter, it typically shows an increased uptake in patients with Graves' disease and toxic multinodular goiter. However, it has been reported that ^{131}I uptake was normal in 27% of elderly patients with Graves' disease and 70% of patients with toxic multinodular goiter.

3. It would be prudent to have a Spanish-speaking psychiatrist evaluate this patient to determine whether any component of dementia or a formal thought disorder was present. In addition, an endocrinologist should be consulted for the immediate and ongoing therapy of the patient's probable hyperthyroidism.

4. Appropriate acute treatment would include the use of a beta blocker for control of adrenergic symptoms. In addition, iodine would help to control her acute symptoms by blocking binding sites for T_4. Propylthiouracil might be an option for acute treatment; its

mechanism of action is that it inhibits organification of iodine and prevents peripheral conversion of T_4 to T_3. However, propylthiouracil is associated with an incidence of agranulocytosis, particularly in persons over the age of 40.

Definitive therapy consists of ablation of the hyperactive gland with ^{131}I. The patient must be controlled symptomatically prior to administration of ^{131}I, because of the transient outpouring of thyroxine at the time of administration. The most common long term side effect of ^{131}I administration is hypothyroidism, which can then be treated with levothyroxine replacement therapy.

5. Hyperthyroidism is characterized by heat intolerance, increased perspiration, tachycardia, palpitations, weight loss despite increased appetite, and diarrhea. However, the manifestations of adrenergic hyperactivity usually seen in younger hyperthyroid patients may be absent in the elderly, to the point where the patient may appear "apathetic."

PEARLS:

1. Elderly patients with hyperthyroidism may be largely free of the manifestations of adrenergic hyperactivity usually seen in this condition in younger people.

2. Thyroid storm (thyrotoxic crisis) is an intensification of the clinical syndrome of thyrotoxicosis. If you suspect thyrotoxic crisis, don't wait for lab results--begin therapy immediately.

3. Thyrotoxic crisis develops most often after a stressful precipitating event such as trauma, infection, surgical emergency, or parturition. Taking a careful history is paramount.

4. Emergency Department screening is not uniformly indicated for patients admitted with acute medical or psychiatric illness, because transient abnormalities may be indistinguishable from true thyroid disease. Testing is most useful if there is clinical suspicion of thyroid disease.

PITFALLS:

1. As patients age, the goiter tends to sit lower in the neck. Frequently, only the most superior aspect of a substernal goiter can be adequately palpated, so it is extremely important to have the patient swallow as you palpate the most inferior aspect of the neck.

2. The diagnosis of thyroid storm must be made clinically--lab results are not significantly different from those in noncritical thyrotoxic patients--and it must be made quickly, because mortality may approach 90% without appropriate therapy.

3. Bear in mind that the precipitating cause of thyroid storm may be masked by the signs and symptoms of thyrotoxic crisis.

REFERENCES:

Bethune JE. Interpretation of thyroid function tests. Dis Mon 1989;35(8):541-595.

Helfand M, Crapo LM. Screening for thyroid disease. Ann Intern Med 1990;112(11):840-849.

Stoffer SS, Szpunar WE. Thyroid disease in the elderly. How is it different than in other age-groups? Postgrad Med 1988;84(6):133-136, 138.

Surks MI, Chopra IJ, Mariash CN, et al. American Thyroid Association guidelines for use of laboratory tests in thyroid disorders. JAMA 1990;263(11):1529-1532.

WRIST PAIN

Case 8:

A 30-year-old attorney presented with pain in his left wrist. The pain began after he fell onto his outstretched left hand during a racquetball game the previous day. The pain was still present when he woke up and was exacerbated with motion. The patient was righthanded and stated that he had never injured either hand or wrist before. He added that he felt it was just a sprain, but wanted x-rays taken. Physical examination was unremarkable except for tenderness to palpation between the tendons of the abductor pollicus longus and extensor pollicus longus.

DIAGNOSTIC CLUE:

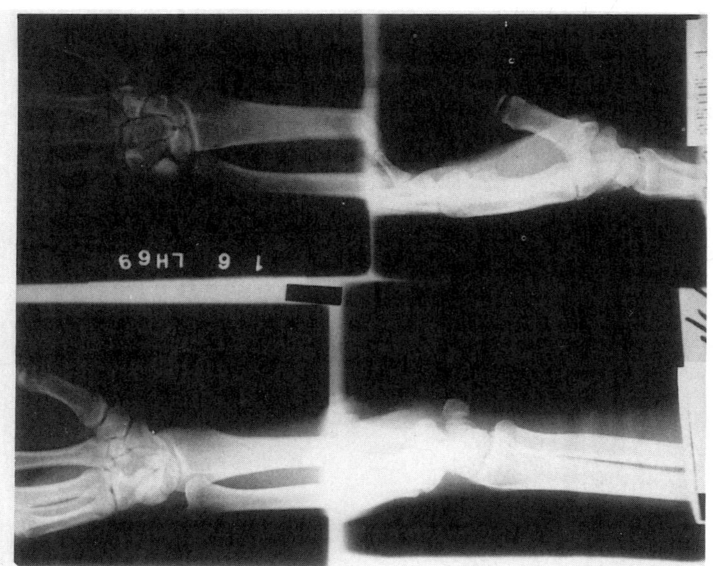

QUESTIONS:

1. What is the diagnosis?

2. Discuss key findings on x-ray examination of the wrist. How many views are necessary?

3. Which findings on the wrist examination are important to document?

4. How should this patient be managed in the ED?

5. What are the complications associated with this injury?

ANSWERS:

1. In order to accurately diagnose traumatic injuries of the wrist, the mechanism of injury must be understood. An accurate history will help focus the physical examination and subsequent radiographic studies.

The most common mechanism of injury to the wrist is seen with a fall on an outstretched hand, forcing the wrist into hyperextension. The scaphoid is particularly susceptible to injury because it bridges the two rows of carpal bones and the radius. In fact, 75% of carpal fractures occur at the scaphoid. Whenever a patient presents with wrist pain after a hyperextension injury of the wrist, a scaphoid fracture must be suspected.

2. A minimum of three views of the wrist should be taken, although special views of the wrist may be necessary in order to view specific injuries. Standard radiographic views include posteroanterior (PA), lateral, and oblique projections. When a scaphoid fracture is suspected, a PA view with the wrist in ulnar deviation and slight flexion is taken; this is known as a scaphoid or navicular view.

On the PA view, first check the integrity of the bony cortices of the eight carpal bones. They are arranged in two rows with the proximal cortices of the proximal carpal row forming a smooth arc. Likewise, the midcarpal joint between the proximal and distal rows should form a smooth crescent. An asymmetric enlargement of a joint space should lead to suspicion of ligamentous instability. For example, an easily missed injury is a scapholunate dislocation or rotary subluxation of the scaphoid, which will appear as a gap greater than 2 mm between the scaphoid and lunate on the PA view.

The lateral view is important in detecting both ligamentous instability and subtle fractures. In a normal lateral view of the wrist, the distal radius, lunate, and proximal portion of the capitate should form three parallel C shapes; a break in the continuity of this pattern indicates an unstable wrist. If the lunate remains in the concavity of the radius but the capitate and remaining carpal bones are displaced this is referred to as a perilunate dislocation. If the lunate is displaced volarly but the remaining bones remain aligned, this is known as a palmar dislocation of the lunate.

A normal PA view foreshortens the scaphoid, but by ulnar deviation and flexion of the wrist, the scaphoid can be seen in full view.

If a high index of suspicion persists despite normal x-rays, it may be necessary to repeat x-rays at a later date (approximately 2 weeks) or to obtain a bone scan, CAT scan, or MRI.

3. Since radiographic studies of the wrist will not always give a definitive answer, it is important to examine the wrist in a methodical manner. This requires familiarity with the topographic anatomy of the wrist.

In general, the physician should document the gross appearance and resting posture of the hand and wrist. This should be followed by having the patient put the wrist through a full range of movement, with pronation and supination being the most important motions. Next, the physician should palpate the various bony landmarks of the wrist in a systematic manner, documenting areas of tenderness and/or crepitation. Do not stop the examination once there is a positive finding--often there may be more than one injury. Finally, one should always document the vascular and neurological integrity of the hand.

When a scaphoid fracture is suspected, as in this case, it is important to palpate the anatomical snuff box. This region is made visible when the thumb is extended and abducted as in hitchhiking. It is the space between the extensor pollices brevis and extensor pollices longus tendons. In addition to tenderness to palpation of the anatomical snuff box, other clues to scaphoid fracture will be pain on gentle ulnar deviation of the pronated hand and pain on axial compression of the thumb (scaphoid compression tenderness).

4. The guiding principle in the management of wrist injuries is to treat on the basis of mechanism of injury and signs on physical examination, rather than on radiographic appearance. Fractures of the scaphoid can be difficult to visualize. For the emergency physician, clinical suspicion of a scaphoid fracture is justification for immobilization. However, there is no universal agreement on the best method of immobilization; some authors advocate a long arm thumb spica cast (above the elbow), incorporating the entire thumb, while the authors of this volume utilize a short arm thumb spica cast from the midpoint of the forearm extending to include the proximal phalanx for clinically suspected scaphoid fractures. No matter what type of immobilization is used, follow-up with a hand specialist in 1 to 2 weeks must be arranged for reexamination.

If there is radiographic evidence of a displaced scaphoid fracture, urgent consultation with a hand specialist is necessary for either an attempted closed reduction or an open reduction. The best chance for restoration of normal wrist function is early restoration of the disrupted anatomy.

5. Avascular necrosis and nonunion are the two main concerns with scaphoid fractures; both can lead to disabling arthritis of the wrist. Problems with healing of scaphoid fractures stem from the tenuous blood supply to the scaphoid bone, which travels distal to proximal. Most fractures of the scaphoid involve the distal or middle third and heal without difficulty if properly treated. Fractures of the proximal third of the scaphoid pose

the greatest risk for nonunion or avascular necrosis. Patients with proximal or displaced scaphoid fractures should be informed of complications at the onset.

PEARLS:

1. Certain mechanisms of injury are associated with specific disorders:
    - Fall on hyperextended wrist (scaphoid fracture)
    - Hypothenar impaction (perilunate dislocation)
    - Closed fist impact (metacarpal fracture)

2. If both active and passive joint motion are impaired, think osseous or ligamentous injury. Normal painless joint motion with absence of active motion suggests tendon disruption.

3. Always compare the injured and noninjured side.

4. A scaphoid fracture should be suspected in every case of an "acutely sprained wrist."

PITFALLS:

1. Do not let the presence of a scaphoid fracture cause you to miss a concomitant scapholunate dislocation or perilunate dislocation.

2. Do not fail to inquire about previous wrist injuries. Even "minor" wrist sprains may be occult scaphoid fractures.

3. Never forget to inform patients that initial readings of x-ray films are preliminary interpretations.

4. Do not fail to appreciate the relationship of the scaphoid and lunate. The normal width between these two carpal bones is 1 to 2 mm in the PA projection. Spaces greater than 2 mm are considered abnormal.

REFERENCES:

DaCruz DJ. The suspected fracture of the scaphoid: a rational approach to the diagnosis. Injury 1988;19:149-155.

Hamlin C. Diagnosis of wrist injuries. Emerg Med Clin North Am 1985;3:311-318.

Hoppenfeld S. Physical examination of the wrist and hand. In: Hoppenfeld S, ed. Physical examination of the spine and extremities. New York: Appleton Century Crofts, 1976:59-104.

Powell JM, Lloyd GJ, Rintoul RF. New clinical test for fracture of the scaphoid. Can J Surg 1988;31:234-238.

Stein F. Radiographic examination of the hand and wrist. Emerg Med Clin North Am 1985;3:221-234.

Young MRA, Lowry JH, McCleod NW, Crome RS. Clinical carpal scaphoid injuries. Br Med J 1988;296:825-826.

AN INTENTIONAL INGESTION

Case 9:

A 35-year-old man was brought to the Emergency Department after taking an unknown amount of Theo-Dur and alcohol during the night. His wife called the paramedics because she noted her husband to be vomiting and shaking in the bathroom. The patient stated that he was depressed and wanted to kill himself.

His past medical history was significant for smoking two packs of cigarettes/day for 20 years. His private physician had started him on Theo-Dur 300 mg twice a day 1 week earlier for "bronchitis." His wife added that he had become increasingly depressed over the past 2 weeks because he was laid off from work.

Upon arrival in the ED, the patient vomited a small quantity of partially digested food. He was slow to answer questions, but knew he was in a hospital. Vital signs on presentation revealed a pulse of 160/minute, respiratory rate of 28/minute, blood pressure of 110/76, and a rectal temperature of 98° F. The remainder of the physical examination was unremarkable.

DIAGNOSTIC CLUES:

Serum theophylline level	86 μg/mL
Serum potassium	2.6 mEq/L
Serum glucose	189 mg%
Serum alcohol level	150 mg%

QUESTIONS:

1. Discuss the initial management of this patient, including the optimal approach for minimizing gastric absorption of ingested theophylline.

2. Is the type of theophylline preparation relevant? How does an acute overdose of theophylline differ from a chronic overdose in terms of toxic serum blood levels and treatment decisions?

3. What factors predispose a patient to theophylline toxicity?

4. What is the role of charcoal hemoperfusion?

ANSWERS:

1. In this case, there is sufficient evidence of severe, toxic theophylline ingestion (viz., protracted vomiting, hypokalemia, tachycardia and serum theophylline level greater than 60 μg/ml) to warrant intervention beyond supportive therapy. Nevertheless, it is important to heed the axiom of treating the patient and not the poison when approaching an overdose patient. Once the patient's airway, breathing, and circulation are stabilized, attention should be directed toward the history, and an attempt should be made to identify the specific toxin. Additionally, any patient with an altered mental status should be given oxygen, naloxone, dextrose, and thiamine as well as be placed on a cardiac monitor.

Another crucial early decision is deciding if the patient will be able to protect his airway. The presence of a gag reflex usually (although not invariably) suggests voluntary presence of airway protection from aspiration. Another axiom to bear in mind is that the overdose patient who can be easily intubated due to depressed gag reflex or mental status probably should be intubated.

In toxicology, the gastrointestinal system assumes a high priority. This is the site through which most toxins are absorbed and therefore the place where most interventions are directed. Traditionally, gastrointestinal decontamination begins with emesis or lavage. Emesis is usually induced with syrup of ipecac, which normally produces results within 30 to 45 minutes. The alternative to emesis is gastric lavage, which utilizes a large bore tube (36 to 40 French), through which 150- to 200-cc aliquots of water or saline are introduced into the gastrointestinal tract and subsequently withdrawn.

There is currently debate on which method of gastrointestinal evacuation is best and when gastrointestinal evacuation is warranted. Each method has its own complications and contraindications. The patient in this case has already vomited, and there is no advantage to induced emesis over "natural" emesis. Moreover, use of ipecac for overdoses of toxins which can provoke seizures (e.g., theophylline, tricyclics) is specifically contraindicated because of the risk of aspiration. Finally, whole bowel irrigation with a polyethylene glycol solution may have a role in overdoses with sustained release preparations who present late.

While treatment of theophylline overdose must be individualized, activated charcoal remains the mainstay of treatment. The charcoal not only binds the remaining theophylline in the gut, but also promotes secretion of absorbed theophylline from the bloodstream back into the gastrointestinal lumen. This back diffusion is known as "gut dialysis." The dose of activated charcoal varies but is usually approximated at 1 g/kg body weight, with an initial dose of 60 g given to most average-sized adults. Most toxicologists concomitantly administer a cathartic such as sorbitol with the first dose of charcoal. The rationale is that charcoal can be constipating and the cathartic will help ensure the passage of the stool and lessen the intestinal transit time of the drug.

Recent work has focused on the use of repeated doses of charcoal as frequently as every 1 to 2 hours. There are reports of continuous nasogastric administration of activated charcoal for theophylline overdoses resulting in significant reduction of serum theophylline levels. As mentioned earlier, the side effects of theophylline toxicity include nausea and vomiting, making charcoal administration difficult. Metoclopramide, antiemetic agents such a promethazine, or the use of a duodenal tube have been advocated to overcome this problem.

There has also been recent interest in the use of beta blockers for treating theophylline overdose. Beta adrenergic stimulation appears responsible for many of the side effects of theophylline toxicity and beta blockerrs such as propranolol and esmolol have been reported to counteract the hypotension (beta-2 mediated) and arrhythmias (beta-1 mediated) associated with theophylline overdose. Caution must be exercised when utilizing these agents in patients with reactive airway disease.

2. Theophylline is one of the most commonly prescribed medications for respiratory disorders. It is available in many forms, including sustained-release products that can maintain constant or increasing levels for 8 to 12 hours or longer. The importance of noting the ingestion of sustained-release products is that the initial serum theophylline level may not reflect the true extent of the ingestion.

Because of the drug's narrow therapeutic index, theophylline intoxication is a common problem. There are usually two distinct clinical syndromes: the single acute overdose versus the chronic overdose. The chronic overdose patient is one who regularly ingests theophylline products, and toxicity results from either incorrect calculation of the dosage on the part of the patient or the physician, or a decreased clearance of theophylline due to congestive heart failure, liver disease or drug interaction.

The patient with an acute overdose will usually present with prominent gastrointestinal symptoms, while the patient who is chronically toxic may demonstrate little if any gastrointestinal disturbance. In addition, in chronic overdoses, there is less correlation between theophylline serum levels and the severity of the overdose. It also appears that patients who have massive single ingestions can better tolerate higher serum theophylline levels than patients who are chronically taking the drug.

3. Theophylline is primarily eliminated by hepatic metabolism utilizing the cytochrome oxidase system. Any disease process which interferes with liver function can protract theophylline breakdown and result in inadvertent theophylline intoxication. Additionally, theophylline metabolism is delayed by numerous other factors, including the presence of congestive heart failure, viral illness such as influenza, and certain medications (cimetidine, ciprofloxacin, and erythromycin). Age has become increasingly recognized as an important variable; the elderly patient has a much slower clearance rate of

theophylline and is much more prone to the life-threatening side effects of theophylline (seizures, arrhythmias, and hypotension) even at lower toxic levels.

4. Hemoperfusion is similar to hemodialysis in that blood is circulated extracorporally, but with hemoperfusion the blood passes through a column filled with an absorbent material such as charcoal. An important parameter which influences the effectiveness of hemoperfusion is the drug's volume of distribution. In general, volume of distribution is a measure of whether a drug is highly tissue soluble (large volume of distribution) or remains confined to the vascular space (small volume of distribution). From a practical standpoint, a drug which has a high volume of distribution is widely distributed and not amenable to hemoperfusion.

Charcoal hemoperfusion has been found to be effective in theophylline overdoses, being up to four to six times more effective than hemodialysis. In general, charcoal hemoperfusion is indicated in patients with life-threatening complications such as status epilepticus, arrhythmias, or hemodynamic instability. Early use of charcoal hemoperfusion should be considered in patients with rapidly rising theophylline levels despite charcoal therapy, in patients with intractable vomiting who cannot keep charcoal down, and in the very old and very young who are theophylline toxic. While some toxicologists quote specific values (e.g., greater than 100 μg/mL in an acute ingestion and greater than 60 μg/mL in a chronic ingestion), it is difficult to substantiate these numbers in controlled studies. In fact, patients with chronic theophylline levels of 40 μg/mL have been known to seize, while patients with acute ingestion values of 190 μg/mL or greater have been known to recover uneventfully. However, once a patient seizes, potential mortality increases dramatically (up to 50%).

Hemoperfusion is not free of problems. Hemoperfusion requires that the patient be anticoagulated, as it may cause platelet depletion and hypocalcemia, conditions which create the potential for bleeding problems. Charcoal hemoperfusion will not correct acid-base, fluid or electrolyte abnormalities. Nevertheless, charcoal hemoperfusion is usually effective in lowering theophylline levels to nontoxic values in the first 2 to 3 hours.

PEARLS:

1. Always treat the patient before the poison.

2. Any overdose patient who is comatose and can tolerate intubation should be intubated.

3. Severe, acute overdoses of theophylline are often associated with hypokalemia, hyperglycemia, hypercalcemia, hypophosphatemia, and metabolic acidosis.

4. Tachycardia is a cardinal manifestation of theophylline intoxication. Lack of a tachycardic response suggests either nontoxic overdose of theophylline or concomitant ingestion of a substance that can slow heart rate.

5. The elderly patient is much more susceptible to life-threatening complications from chronic theophylline overdose than the younger patient.

PITFALLS:

1. Do not fail to ensure airway protection.

2. Do not rely on premonitory symptoms to predict seizures. They are particularly unreliable in chronic overdoses.

3. Do not administer ipecac to a patient who is comatose, or seizing, or has lost the protective airway reflexes or may lose airway reflexes in the next 45 minutes. Also remember that ipecac can delay administration of life-saving therapy such as charcoal.

4. Never rely on initial serum theophylline levels. A second theophylline level allows the physician to determine if more theophylline is being absorbed, particularly with sustained-release preparations.

5. Remember to obtain psychiatric clearance on all intentional overdose patients.

REFERENCES:

Aitken ML, Martin TR: Life threatening toxicity is not predictable by serum levels. Chest 1987;91:10-14.

Katona BG, Siegel EG, Cluxton RJ: The new black magic: activated charcoal and new therapeutic uses. J Emerg Med 1987;5:9-18.

Olson KR, Benowitz NL, Woo OF, et al: Theophylline overdose: acute single ingestion versus chronic repeated overmedication. Am J Emerg Med 1985;3:386-394.

Paloucek FP, Rodvold KA: Evaluation of theophylline overdoses and toxicities. Ann Emerg Med 1988;17:135-144.

A CONFUSED NURSING HOME RESIDENT

Case 10:

An 87-year-old white female was transferred to the Emergency Department from a nursing home. The patient was unable to give any history; however, the nursing home summary sheet indicated that she was referred for a fever of 102° F for 2 days with decreased responsiveness. The patient was said to be moderately demented at baseline, but apparently was normally ambulatory. The summary did not state if the patient had complained of any specific symptoms or exhibited any localizing signs since the onset of the fever. There was no history of recent trauma. Her past medical history was significant for multiinfarct dementia diagnosed 6 years earlier, noninsulin dependent diabetes mellitus for 20 years, osteoarthritis for 20 years, hypertension for 20 years, peripheral vascular disease for 15 years, and congestive heart failure for 10 years. The patient's medications included Diabinese 250 mg daily, ibuprofen 400 mg qid, methyldopa 250 mg tid, pentoxyphylline 400 mg tid, diisorbide nitrate 10 mg qid, nitroglycerin 1/150 SL PRN, digoxin 0.250 mg daily, furosemide 40 mg daily, and potassium chloride 20 mEq daily. There was no known history of allergies, smoking, or alcohol abuse.

She was a cachectic elderly female who appeared agitated, making loud repetitive incoherent sounds an pulling at her sheets. Her blood pressure was 90/50, her pulse was 110/minute and regular, her respiratory rate was 28/minute, and her temperature was 102.4° F rectally. Her head was atraumatic. Extraocular movements were intact, with anicteric conjunctivae and equal and reactive pupils. Her ocular fundi were not visualized due to bilateral cataracts. Her tympanic membranes were not visualized due to dense cerumen bilaterally. Her dentition was very poor. Her neck was resistant to movement in all directions, with no adenopathy and no thyromegaly. The carotids were 1+ bilaterally with normal upstrokes and no bruits. Her lung exam revealed bibasilar rales posteriorly with a poor inspiratory effort. Her heart exam was notable for a normal S1 and S2 with an intermittent S3 and a grade II/VI systolic ejection nonradiating murmur at the base, without any rub. Her abdomen was soft and nontender with hypoactive bowel sounds. The liver span was 8 cm, and there was no splenomegaly or mass. Rectal exam revealed heme-negative hard stool. Her extremities were notable for moderate bilateral pedal edema and absent posterior tibialis and dorsalis pedis pulses bilaterally. Diffuse osteoarthritic joint changes were noted. On neurologic exam, the patient was found to be responsive to pain, but not clearly responsive to verbal stimuli. She moved all extremities freely. Sensory function, cerebellar function, and gait could not be ascertained with accuracy. Deep tendon reflexes were moderately diminished diffusely. Her skin was notable for mottling over her lower extremities and purpuric lesions scattered over her trunk.

DIAGNOSTIC CLUES:

CBC:

White blood cell count = 24,600
Hematocrit = 28.4%
Platelet count = 104,000

SMA:

Sodium = 133
Potassium = 5.3
Chloride = 97
Bicarbonate = 20
Glucose = 287
BUN = 45
Creatinine = 1.8

Urinalysis:

Unremarkable

Cerebrospinal fluid:

Leukocytes = 8,600 cells/cu mm, with 80% polymorphonuclear cells
Erythrocytes = 100 cells/cu mm
Glucose = 33
Protein = 162

Gram stain cerebrospinal fluid:

Numerous polymorphonuclear leukocytes with occasional Gram-negative intracellular debris

QUESTIONS:

1. What is the diagnosis?
2. What is the appropriate therapy?
3. What is the patient's prognosis?
4. Should a discussion of resuscitation status be initiated in the Emergency Department?
5. Should prophylactic antibiotic therapy be given to the Emergency Department staff?

ANSWERS:

1. This patient demonstrates the clinical syndrome of meningococcal meningitis. Neisseria meningitidis is the second most common cause of bacterial meningitis in the United States. Endemic meningococcal disease tends to peak from late winter to early spring. The incidence of meningococcal disease is believed to be highest among children 6 to 12 months of age. Patients with immune compromise are also at increased risk, particularly persons with chronic conditions such as asplenia and complement deficiency. The diagnosis may be made in the Emergency Department on Gram stain of cerebrospinal fluid, with findings being a predominance of polymorphonuclear cells and the presence of characteristic Gram-negative diplococci. Unfortunately, diplococci may be rare and in over 50% of cases are difficult to distinguish on Gram stain of either a spun or unspun specimen. In most cases, the diagnosis is made on clinical evaluation.

Meningococcal meningitis should always be suspected:

a. In epidemics of meningitis
b. When the evolution of meningitis is extremely rapid
c. When the onset is accompanied by a morbilliform, petechial, or purpuric skin eruption; large ecchymoses; and lividity of the skin of lower parts of the body
d. If circulatory collapse has occurred

Since a rash accompanies approximately 50% of meningococcal infections, its presence should dictate immediate institution of therapy for a neisserial infection, even though similar rashes may be observed with viral and other bacterial meningitides.

Fulminant meningococcemia with adrenocortical necrosis (the Waterhouse-Friderichsen syndrome) is associated with vasomotor collapse and shock. The onset is abrupt, and profound prostration frequently occurs within a few hours. Petechiae and purpuric lesions enlarge rapidly, and hemorrhage into the skin may be extensive. In the preshock stage, patients are alert and pale, with circumoral cyanosis and cold extremities due to generalized vasoconstriction. Evolution of frank shock is usually accompanied by coma, decreased cardiac output, and hypotension.

2. Therapy should be instituted as soon as meningococcal disease is suspected. Penicillin G is the drug of choice and should be administered intravenously as 12 to 24 million units/day for adults. Meningococci are susceptible to other antimicrobial agents such as chloramphenicol and tetracycline, but these should not be used unless a patient is allergic to penicillin. In patients over age 60 who have a nondiagnostic cerebrospinal fluid, other Gram-negative organisms are a consideration. Empiric therapy should include ampicillin or a third-generation cephalosporin plus gentamicin.

Patients with meningococcal infections require supportive treatment as well as antimicrobial therapy. Maintenance of fluid and electrolyte balance and prevention of respiratory complications in comatose patients are of primary concern. Shock must be treated aggressively.

3. The mortality rate of meningococcal meningitis is between 5 and 15%. The prognosis is worsened by the presence of old age or infancy, abrupt onset, bacteremia, coma, seizures, or such concomitant diseases as alcoholism, diabetes mellitus, and multiple myeloma. Additional findings which appear to be associated with a worsened prognosis include acidosis, thrombocytopenia, hypoglycemia, and serum white blood cell count. Meningococcemia is associated with a somewhat higher fatality rate because of the fulminant nature of the disease and the complications of adrenocortical necrosis and shock.

4. Resuscitation status is certainly a topic which should be addressed promptly in this critically ill patient. Since this patient was admitted from a nursing home, there exists the possibility that a living will or health care proxy or the equivalent were executed upon admission to the nursing home. This practice has become increasingly common and is now required upon admission to many skilled nursing facilities.

5. A great deal of anxiety and even hysteria surrounds prophylactic therapy of hospital personnel with possible exposure to meningococcal meningitis. Once the physician ascertains that the risk of meningococcal disease exists in a patient, the first step is to place the patient in respiratory isolation in the Emergency Department. Respiratory isolation procedures simply require that the patient be placed in a private room and that masks be worn. The second step is to immediately contact the Infection Control or Infectious Disease department of the hospital. This will ensure that appropriate guidelines are followed for detection of personnel at risk and correct prophylaxis is prescribed.

In general, hospital personnel eligible for prophylaxis after exposure to meningococcal meningitis include

- a. Those involved in mouth-to-mouth resuscitation
- b. Those involved in intubation of the patient
- c. Those who performed an oral or funduscopic examination
- d. Those who assisted a vomiting patient
- e. Those on whom the patient has breathed directly

Antimicrobial prophylaxis after exposure to meningococcal meningitis consists of rifampin 600 mg orally twice a day for 2 days.

PEARLS:

1. Patients with bacterial meningitis should have x-rays of the chest, skull, and sinuses as soon as possible after admission. Chest films may reveal pneumonitis or abscess, and sinus and skull films may provide clues to the presence of cranial osteomyelitis, paranasal sinusitis, or mastoiditis.

2. Meningococci may be demonstrated on Gram stain of material aspirated from nodular petechiae or the buffy coat of blood from patients with meningococcemia.

PITFALLS:

1. Failure to recognize incipient shock in a patient with meningococcal infection will almost invariably result in the patient's death.

2. Although bacterial meningitis typically results in a polymorphonuclear leukocytosis of the cerebrospinal fluid, it is possible to see a predominantly lymphocytic response early in the course of infection as well as in immunocompromised hosts.

3. Failure to follow appropriate Infection Control guidelines in prophylaxis of exposed personnel can result in unnecessary hysteria, potentially dangerous complications of unnecessary therapy, and inadequate detection of exposed personnel.

REFERENCES:

Arevalo CE, Barnes PF, Duda M, Leedom JM. Cerebrospinal fluid cell counts and chemistries in bacterial meningitis. South Med J 1989;82(9):1122-1127.

Emparanza JI, Aldamiz-Echevarria L, Perez-Yarza EG, et al. Prognostic score in acute meningococcemia. Crit Care Med 1988;16(2):168-169.

Gillum JE, Garrison MW, Crossley KB, Rotschafer JC. Current immunization practices. Postgrad Med 1989;85(2):199-202, 207-210.

Gurevich I. Transmissible infections in critical care. Heart Lung 1988;17(4):331-334.

Marton KI, Gean AD. The spinal tap: a new look at an old test. Ann Int Med 1986;104:840-848.

AN AGITATED MAN BROUGHT IN BY THE POLICE

Case 11:

An agitated and combative white male who appeared to be in his forties was brought to the Emergency Department by police, who found him staggering down the middle of a local highway, gesticulating and yelling incoherently while removing his clothing. He was alone, and no further medical history could be obtained.

On examination, the patient was tossing restlessly on a stretcher, with temporary wrist and leg restraints. He was diaphoretic and tremulous and entirely uncooperative. His speech was garbled and slurred. His clothing was torn and dirty. There was no evidence of alcohol on his breath. His blood pressure was 140/90, his pulse was 110/minute and regular, his respiratory rate was 16/minute, and his temperature was 98.8° F rectally. His head was atraumatic. His extraocular movements were intact; pupils were round, regular, and reactive to light; and his conjunctivae were anicteric. His oral hygiene appeared poor with poor dentition. He moved his neck spontaneously in all directions. No thyromegaly was palpable.

Lungs were clear bilaterally. His heart sounds were normal, with no murmur or gallop appreciated. His abdomen was nontender, with normal bowel sounds and diffuse guarding. Organ size could not be assessed. He had several tatoos on his upper extremities, with bilateral Dupuytren's contractures of his hands. There were no track marks seen, and no evidence of cyanosis or edema. Neurologic examination was difficult. His motor and sensory function appeared grossly normal. He would not cooperate for cranial nerve or cerebellar exam, although no gross deficits were observed.
An intravenous line was started with D5W at a rate of 50 cc/hour and the following laboratory tests ordered. The patient was treated with pentobarbital 50 mg IM for presumed ethanol withdrawal.

DIAGNOSTIC CLUES:

Hematocrit: 47%
Serum white blood cells: 9800 with normal differential count
Sodium: 150
Potassium: 4.4
BUN: 20
Calcium: 8.5
Chloride: 112
Bicarbonate: 30
Creatinine: 1.9
Glucose: 24
Serum amylase: 60
Serum ethanol level: None detected
Urinalysis: No white cells, red cells, or protein; ketones 1+

QUESTIONS:

1. What mistake in the diagnostic process was made here?

2. What mistake in therapy was made here?

3. What is the appropriate diagnosis?

4. What is the appropriate therapy?

5. What are potential sequelae of delayed treatment for this patient?

ANSWERS:

1. A critical error was made when the patient's serum glucose was overlooked. An immediate lab stick for glucose should be peformed on all Emergency Department patients who present with a change in mental status. The patient's glucose was 24, indicating severe hypoglycemia. Diaphoresis, tremulousness, and tachycardia can be symptoms of either ethanol withdrawal or hypoglycemia. Moreover, alcoholics can become hypoglycemic as well as be in alcoholic withdrawal. Although the patient had bilateral Dupuytren's contractures, which can be seen in association with chronic alcohol abuse, there is no other evidence to indicate that he was an ethanol abuser.

2. The patient with presumed hypoglycemia should receive sufficient glucose repletion. This patient should have received 50 cc of D50 as an intravenous bolus for immediate relief of his hypoglycemia. An intravenous drip of 50 cc/hour of D5W would not reverse his hypoglycemia rapidly enough.

Second, alcoholics or patients suspected of being alcohol abusers should never be given intravenous glucose without prior or concomitant administration of thiamine. Glucose enters the Krebs cycle, utilizing thiamine pyrophosphate. In the thiamine-depleted alcoholic, a glucose bolus can result in acute thiamine deficiency (Wernicke's syndrome, in which symptoms include ophthalmoplegia, nystagmus, ataxia, and confusion.)

3. The appropriate diagnosis is acute hypoglycemia. Patients at risk for acute hypoglycemia include diabetics who take their insulin and do not eat or incorrectly administer an excessive dose of insulin. Noninsulin dependent diabetics may present with hypoglycemia due to oral hypoglycemic agents, which may occur through inadvertent overdosage or lack of eating. Elderly patients, whose body composition includes an increased percentage of body fat, may develop a large reservoir of lipid-soluble oral hypoglycemics; these patients may present with a profound and prolonged hypoglycemia which can last for days.

Alcoholics can become hypoglycemic from poor nutrition as well as diminished glycogen stores secondary to chronic hepatic insufficiency. The metabolism of ethanol uses up NAD, thereby depleting stores necessary for gluconeogenesis. In addition, alcohol abuse can lead to chronic pancreatitis with pancreatic insufficiency and diabetes. These individuals become insulin dependent and may become acutely hypoglycemia from either incorrect administration of insulin or taking insulin without eating.

Common causes of hypoglycemia include the following:

I. Fasting hypoglycemia
   A. Underproduction of glucose by the liver
      1. Acquired liver disease (hepatitis, cirrhosis, congestive heart failure)
      2. Drugs (ethanol, propranolol, salicylates)
      3. Amino acid substrate deficiency (malnutrition, chronic renal failure)
   B. Overutilization of glucose
      1. Exogenous insulin administration (most common cause of hypoglycemia)
      2. Sulfonylurea ingestion
      3. Insulinoma

II. Postprandial hypoglycemia
   A. Rapid gastric emptying (prior gastrectomy, gastrojejunostomy, or pyloroplasty)
   B. Idiopathic postprandial hypoglycemia

4. Appropriate therapy for hypoglycemia consists of one 50 cc ampule of D50 as an intravenous bolus. If the patient does not respond, a second ampule can be given. As soon as the patient regains normal consciousness and is no longer symptomatic, the intravenous boluses can be replaced by an intravenous drip, initially of D10W. When two consecutive serum glucoses 1 hour apart are within the normal range, the patient can be switched to D5W, with close monitoring of serum glucose.

5. Untreated hypoglycemia can lead to a wide variety of presenting complaints, include focal neurologic deficits, focal seizures, isolated aglossia, and acute violent behavior. Hypoglycemia should always be suspected with any case of altered mental status, neurologic abnormality, or bizarre behavior.

Symptoms of hypoglycemia can be divided into adrenergic and central nervous system "neuroglycopenic" symptoms. Adrenergic symptoms tend to have a more sudden onset and are typically postprandial complaints. These include anxiety, irritability, palpitations, sweating, tachycardia, and tremor. Neuroglycopenic symptoms often have a more gradual onset and are typically fasting complaints. These include headache, fatigue, hypothermia, confusion, amnesia, seizures, loss of consciousness, irrational behavior, a glassy-eyed stare, diplopia, and dysarthria. Severe hypoglycemia can result in coma and death.

PEARLS:

1. Do not give patients with hepatic insufficiency continued intravenous glucose, since hepatic glycogen stores cannot be repleted with intravenous glucose. Oral intake of glucose is critical.

2. Patients with quickly relieved hypoglycemia who can supply a very cogent reason for the acute episode do not need to be admitted.

PITFALLS:

1. Do not discharge patients with serious or life-threatening symptoms of hypoglycemia, persistent hypoglycemia, or hypoglycemia due to hepatic disease; alcoholics on insulin; patients who have taken long-acting oral hypoglycemic agents; or patients without sufficient social supports to prevent recurrent hypoglycemia.

2. Never assume a diagnosis based on a patient's appearance or behavior. Rule out organic disease in every case.

REFERENCES:

Blackman JD, Towle VL, Lewis GF, et al. Hypoglycemic thresholds for cognitive dysfunction in humans. Diabetes 1990;39(7):828-835.

Felicetta JV. When to worry about hypoglycemia. Postgrad Med 1990;88(1):175-180.

Odeh M, Oliven A, Bassan H. Transient atrial fibrillation precipitated by hypoglycemia. Ann Emerg Med 1990;19(5):565-567.

Weston C, Stephans M. Hypoglycaemic attacks treated by ambulance personnel with extended training. Br Med J 1990;300(6729):908-909.

A WOMAN WITH RECURRENT SEIZURES

Case 12:

A 35-year-old white female was brought to the Emergency Department by ambulance. Her husband stated she had had seizures since childhood and was on seizure medications. She had had no seizures in the past 5 years, and had recently become careless about taking her medications. Approximately 1 hour earlier, she had told her husband she felt strange and had fallen to the floor, shaking all over, and urinating upon herself. Her husband called the ambulance immediately. While they were waiting for the ambulance, she had two more seizures, and she had another two on the way to the hospital. Her usual medications were diphenylhydantoin and phenobarbital, but her husband did not know the doses. She had no other medical history and was taking no other medication. She used no recreational drugs and never drank alcohol.

On examination, she was a well-developed white female lying quietly on the stretcher, breathing deeply and unresponsive except to deep pain. Her blood pressure was 130/80, her pulse was 90/minute and regular, her respiratory rate was 24/minute and regular, and her rectal temperature was 98.8° F. Her head was atraumatic. Her pupils were dilated symmetrically, with flat disks bilaterally. Her tympanic membranes were normal in appearance. Her tongue had a small laceration on the left side. Her neck was supple without thyromegaly or adenopathy. Her lungs were clear bilaterally, and her heart sounds were normal without murmurs, clicks, or gallops. Her abdomen was soft and nontender, with normal bowel sounds and no organomegaly. As the physician began to examine her extremities, she began to seize again, moving her extremities in tonic-clonic movements.

DIAGNOSTIC CLUES:

Dextrostik glucose: 120
SMA6: Pending
CBC: Pending
Diphenylhydantoin level: Pending
Phenobarbital level: Pending

QUESTIONS:

1. How is status epilepticus defined?

2. What are possible causes of status epilepticus?

3. What is the natural history of status epilepticus?

4. What is the appropriate therapy for this patient?

ANSWERS:

1. Status epilepticus has been defined as a state in which seizures are of sufficient length or are repeated frequently enough to produce a fixed and lasting epileptic condition. From a practical standpoint, status epilepticus may be identified as a seizure lasting more than 30 minutes or several distinct episodes without restoration of consciousness.

The classification of status epilepticus is outlined below. Any type of epileptic seizure can develop into status epilepticus, but some types of seizures evolve into status more commonly than others.

Generalized status epilepticus

- Convulsive
  - Tonic
  - Clonic
  - Myoclonic
- Nonconvulsive
  - Absence

Partial status epilepticus

- Simple
  - Somatomotor
  - Aphasic
- Complex
  - Complex partial seizures

The syndrome most commonly associated with the term "status epilepticus" is tonic-clonic or convulsive status epilepticus. In this form, which is most often seen in adults, seizures are either generalized at onset or may be secondarily generalized from partial seizures.

2. Status epilepticus occurs in up to 60,000 individuals in the United States annually. In one-third of cases, status epilepticus is the presenting symptom in patients with a first unprovoked seizure; in another third of cases, epilepsy is established; in the final third, there is no history of epilepsy. The greatest number of cases will occur in children, although the risk is equally high in adults over age 60.

Causes of tonic-clonic status epilepticus include the following:

a. Patients with a background of epilepsy
   - Poor anticonvulsant compliance
   - Recent dose reduction or discontinuation
   - Alcohol withdrawal
   - Pseudostatus

b. Patients with no background of epilepsy
   - Cerebrovascular disease
   - Meningoencephalitis
   - Acute head injury
   - Cerebral tumor
   - Brain abscess
   - Metabolic disorders (renal failure, hypoglycemia, hyponatremia, hepatic encephalopathy, etc.)
   - Drug overdose (tricyclic antidepressants, phenothiazines, theophylline, isoniazid, cocaine)
   - Inflammatory arteritis (systemic lupus erythematosus)

The mortality rate reported with status epilepticus varies from 1 to 10%. However, it appears that mortality is largely related to the underlying cause rather than to the recurrent seizures.

3. Convulsive status epilepticus can lead to hyperthermia, peripheral leukocytosis, pleocytosis, hemodynamic alterations, and respiratory defects, including pulmonary edema. Convulsive status epilepticus is associated with acidosis, changes in blood sugar, and elevation of serum catecholamines, alterations that are important because they can pose a threat to the patient's life. It has been reported that status epilepticus can result in long-term cognitive deficits and decline in intellectual capacity.

The cardiovascular system is particularly stressed because of the excessive demands placed upon it by repeated tonic contractions of the skeletal muscle system. Tachycardia is inevitable; bradycardia may occur because of vagal tone modulated by CNS activity, and cardiac arrhythmias may occur as a result of hyperkalemia. Anticonvulsant drugs may add to these effects, since phenytoin and its solvent propylene glycol may cause arrhythmias and hypotension and barbiturates are myocardial depressants.

Since tonic-clonic seizure is usually followed by great respiratory effort stimulated by hypercapnia, respiratory failure may occur following a series of seizures. Respiratory drive may also be depressed by the disorder, precipitating status epilepticus as well as by the barbiturates and benzodiazepines used for treatment. Changes in lymphatic flow may induce pulmonary edema. Rhabdomyolysis causes myoglobinuria and may result in renal failure.

Massive activation of both sympathetic and parasympathetic systems during status epilepticus leads to severe autonomic nervous system disturbances, including hyperpyrexia, excessive sweating, and salivary and tracheobronchial hypersecretion. Associated endocrine abnormalities include marked elevations in plasma prolactin, glucagon, growth hormone, and adrenocorticotropic hormone.

4. Time is of the essence in the treatment of status epilepticus. The longer the seizures continue, the harder it is to terminate seizure activity. In addition, patients with status epilepticus require constant ongoing surveillance.

There is some controversy regarding the use of phenytoin versus a benzodiazepine as the first-line agent. Advantages of phenytoin include its effectiveness in controlling convulsions, its relatively long half-life, and its lack of significant CNS depression. Disadvantages include its cardiovascular toxicity if given too rapidly, the time required for giving the full loading dose, and its relative ineffectiveness in suppressing focal epileptic activity. Blood pressure and electrocardiogram results <u>must</u> be monitored during <u>slow</u> administration of intravenous phenytoin.

The primary advantage of diazepam is its rapid onset of activity due to quick distribution to the brain. Disadvantages are its tendency to depress respiration and consciousness and its short duration of action and redistribution from the CNS, which limits its effectiveness to less than 30 minutes. Diazepam should be used in conjunction with or be followed by phenytoin loading.

Lorazepam, a longer acting benzodiazepine, has been advocated for the treatment of status epilepticus because of its longer CNS action.

Phenobarbital has the advantage of a very long half-life. It can be administered more rapidly than phenytoin and is effective in generalized and partial seizures. The disadvantage is depression of consciousness and respiration. The depression of respiration may be more profound in a patient who was initially treated with diazepam. The usual starting dose is 10 mg/kg, followed by an additional 10 mg/kg if needed.

Pentobarbital coma has been successfully utilized in status epilepticus refractory to diazepam, phenytoin, and other drugs. Its use should be carefully monitored by EEG recording, and doses should be tailored to maintain a burst-suppression pattern on the EEG. Pentobarbital coma may be required for many days.

Valproic acid has been given rectally for the treatment of status epilepticus. A major disadvantage is its slow absorption relative to drugs that are given intravenously. An intravenous preparation of valproic acid may soon become available; its effectiveness in status epilepticus will need to be assessed.

Time	Intervention
1-5 min	Assess airway, remove false teeth. Assess cardiopulmonary status. Obtain history and perform neurologic and physical examination. Check for signs of head trauma. Insert oral airway and give oxygen if needed.
5-10 min	Establish venous access and draw blood for antiepileptic drug levels, glucose, blood urea nitrogen, electrolytes, metabolic screen, and drug screen. Check glucose at bedside. Start IV saline and administer glucose and thiamine. Immediately administer lorazepam 4 to 8 mg (at a rate of <2 mg/minute IV bolus) or diazepam 10 to 20 mg.
10-40 min	Place patient on cardiac monitor. Begin infusion of phenytoin 20 mg/kg at a rate no faster than 50 mg/minute. Monitor blood pressure and EKG. If seizures persist, give an additional 5 mg/kg and if necessary another 5 mg/kg until a maximum dose of 30 mg/kg is administered.
40-60 min	If seizures persist, intubate the patient and give phenobarbital 20 mg/kg IV push at a rate <100 mg/minute.
60 min	If seizures persist, barbiturate coma or general anesthesia (using agents with which the staff is familiar) should be started.

PEARLS:

1. The more protracted the seizures, the more difficult they are to control.

2. Always search for the underlying cause for status epilepticus, as this is the primary prognostic factor.

3. Protracted status epilepticus is more likely to have protracted effects.

PITFALLS:

1. Status epilepticus due to tricyclic antidepressant overdose may display hypotension as a cardinal feature. Use of phenytoin or barbiturates may accentuate hypotension.

2. Never give phenytoin intravenously any faster than 50 mg/minute. More rapid administration can cause sudden death due to cardiac arrhythmias.

3. Keep watching the patient with status epilepticus closely, even after seizures seem to have stopped.

4. Do not treat status epilepticus with diazepam alone. Its half-life is too short to prevent seizure recurrence.

5. Do not use neuromuscular paralyzing agents, as these will not stop seizure activity in the brain and will make it difficult to assess response to treatment.

REFERENCES:

Brodie MJ. Status epilepticus in adults. Lancet 1990;336(8709):231-234.

Hauser WA. Status epilepticus: epidemiologic considerations. Neurology 1990;40(5 Suppl 2):9-13.

Leppik IE. Status epilepticus: the next decade. Neurology 1990;40(5 Suppl 2):4-9.

Lothman E. The biochemical basis and pathophysiology of status epilepticus. Neurology 1990;40(5 Suppl 2):1-51.

Scheuer ML, Pedley TA. The evaluation and treatment of seizures. New Engl J Med 1990; 323(21): 1468-1474.

AN ELDERLY MAN WITH RECTAL BLEEDING

Case 13:

A 72-year-old male presented complaining of one episode of bloody diarrhea several hours earlier. The patient had been in his usual state of health until the day before, when he noted a "crampy, uncomfortable" feeling in his lower abdomen. The sensation persisted for several hours, but resolved spontaneously. He had no further symptoms until the next day when he noted crampy lower abdominal pain followed by a single episode of loose stool mixed with red blood. He had no nausea, vomiting, constipation, fever, or rectal pain. He denied any previous history of rectal bleeding, hemorrhoids, or gastrointestinal disease. He denied any change in diet, recent travel, or weight loss. His past medical history was significant for hypertension for 10 years, a heart murmur noted 5 years earlier, and osteoarthritis for the past 5 years. His medications included hydrochlorothiazide 50 mg daily, potassium chloride 10 mEq daily, and ibuprofen 400 mg every 4 hours as needed for pain. He had no allergies, had never smoked, and had drunk alcohol sparingly throughout his life.

On examination, he was a well-nourished elderly male in no apparent distress, sitting comfortably on the examining table. His blood pressure was 165/90 and his pulse was 80 and regular, both lying and standing. His respiratory rate was 20/minute and an oral temperature was 98.2° F. Examination of his head and neck was unremarkable. His lungs were clear bilaterally. Auscultation of his heart revealed a normal S1 with a slightly decreased S2 and a low-pitched grade II/VI systolic ejection murmur at the base which radiated faintly into the carotids. The carotid pulses were 2+ bilaterally with normal upstrokes. Auscultation of the abdomen revealed normal bowel sounds in all four quadrants, with no bruits. His abdomen was soft, with mild left lower quadrant tenderness. There were no masses and no evidence of ascites. His liver span was 8 cm, with a soft, nontender edge, and his spleen was not palpable. Rectal exam revealed a small external hemorrhoid which was nontender and did not appear to be bleeding, a nontender prostate of normal size and consistency, and loose brown stool which was strongly heme positive. His extremities were not cyanotic and he had no peripheral edema. His pulses were 2+ diffusely, and he had no adenopathy.

DIAGNOSTIC CLUE:

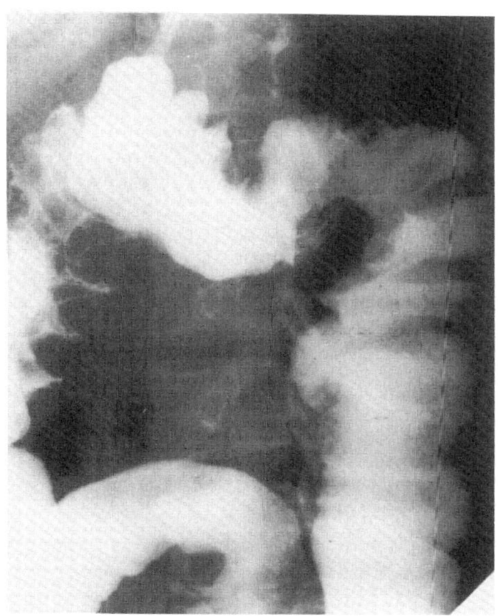

QUESTIONS:

1. What are the most common causes of rectal bleeding in the elderly?

2. Is this patient's heart murmur of any significance to his rectal bleeding?

3. What diagnosis is suggested by his x-ray?

4. Does this man need to be admitted?

5. What would be an appropriate diagnostic plan for lower gastrointestinal bleeding in an elderly patient?

ANSWERS:

1. The most common sources of lower gastrointestinal bleeding in the elderly are diverticula and vascular ectasias, each of which accounts for about 40% of cases. About 20% of bleeding episodes are caused by polyps, internal hemorrhoids, colorectal cancer, radiation-induced colitis, stercoral ulcer, and ischemic colitis. Of this group, ischemic colitis is the most common.

2. There is an association between aortic stenosis and vascular ectasias. Vascular ectasias (also called arteriovenous malformations or angiodysplastic lesions) are found in the cecum and ascending colon of roughly 25% of patients over age 60. These lesions are degenerative and are usually less than 5 mm in diameter. Approximately half of patients with ectasias have heart disease, and 50% of these have aortic stenosis. It is not thought that aortic stenosis increases the incidence of ectasias, but that the low perfusion pressure seen with aortic stenosis may cause ischemic necrosis of the endothelium separating ectatic vessels from the colonic lumen.

3. The x-ray is diagnostic of ischemic colitis, as evidenced by the "thumbprinting" indicative of colonic submucosal edema. Ischemic colitis is seen almost exclusively in the elderly, and this patient's presentation is typical. Any part of the colon can be affected, but most commonly involved are the splenic flexure and the descending and sigmoid colon. The bleeding usually stops spontaneously, and the patient may recover completely, or go on to develop segmental colitis and stricture. Severe cases of ischemia may go on to gangrene and perforation.

4. Since it is not clear whether this patient's ischemia will worsen or resolve, it would be prudent to admit him for continued observation and further diagnostic workup. Since bleeding usually stops spontaneously in ischemic colitis, he can be put at bedrest and placed NPO, with further evaluation performed electively.

5. The first step in diagnosis of hematochezia in the elderly is a careful digital rectal examination. The next step is usually a plain film of the abdomen, if ischemic colitis is suspected. Sigmoidoscopy may reveal a rectal mass or tear, bleeding hemorrhoids, polyps, or distal colitis, and is particularly important in diagnosis of lower gastrointestinal bleeding that is not hemodynamically significant. If bleeding stops promptly or continues slowly, colonoscopy will allow direct visualization of lesions and potential treatment (e.g., removal of polyps, electrocoagulation of ectasias).

Very brisk lower gastrointestinal bleeding suggests an upper gastrointestinal source, and upper endoscopy should be considered. If this is negative a technetium 99m-labeled red cell scan (blood pool scan) may localize the bleeding site. If the scan is positive and colonoscopy is not possible or if both the scan and colonoscopy are negative but bleeding persists, angiography is necessary to look at the superior and inferior mesenteric arteries and celiac trunk.

PEARLS:

1. Upper gastrointestinal bleeding is the third most common cause of brisk rectal bleeding, after ectasias and diverticula.

2. It was previously held that although most diverticula are left sided, most of those that bleed are right sided. It is now felt that much of that right sided bleeding is actually due to vascular ectasias, not diverticula.

PITFALLS:

1. Avoid barium enemas in evaluating acute rectal bleeding, since the barium makes it difficult to carry out subsequent colonoscopy or angiography.

2. Although abdominal pain followed by bleeding is the typical presentation of ischemic colitis, bleeding can precede any other sign or symptom.

REFERENCES:

Boley SJ, Brandt LJ. Vascular ectasias of the colon--1986. Dig Dis Sci 1986;31(suppl 9):2655-4255.

Brandt LJ. Gastrointestinal disorders of the elderly. New York: Raven Press, 1984.

Jhangiani S, Pitchumoni CS. Gastrointestinal bleeding in elderly patients. Comprehensive Therapy 1987;13(5):17-25.

Rosen AM, Fleischer DE. Lower GI bleeding: updated diagnosis and management. Geriatrics 1989;44:49-60.

<u>A MIDDLE-AGED FEMALE WITH CHEST PAIN</u>

Case 14:

A 46-year-old female presented to the nurse at the triage desk complaining of tightness in her chest. She stated she was bitten on the forearm approximately one-half hour prior to presentation by a "bee," and pointed to an area of swelling on her forearm approximately 7 cm in diameter. Shortly, thereafter she related feeling flushed, experiencing nasal stuffiness and developing a "tight" feeling in her chest. Her past medical history was significant for mitral valve prolapse, and the triage note stated that she had presented to the Emergency Department five times in the last 3 months with chest pain. The patient added that her doctor had placed her on propranolol 40 mg twice/day 1 month ago. Other than seasonal allergies, she related no previous allergic history for bee stings or medication.

Her initial vital signs were blood pressure 92/58, pulse 66/minute and regular, respiratory rate 22/minute and slightly labored with faintly audible wheezing and an oral temperature of 98.6° F Her physical examination was notable for faint wheezing over both lung fields posteriorly. Her heart sounds were normal, with an intermittent midsystolic click. Her abdominal examination was unremarkable. Her skin color was fair, with a "rash" noted on the trunk.

DIAGNOSTIC CLUES:

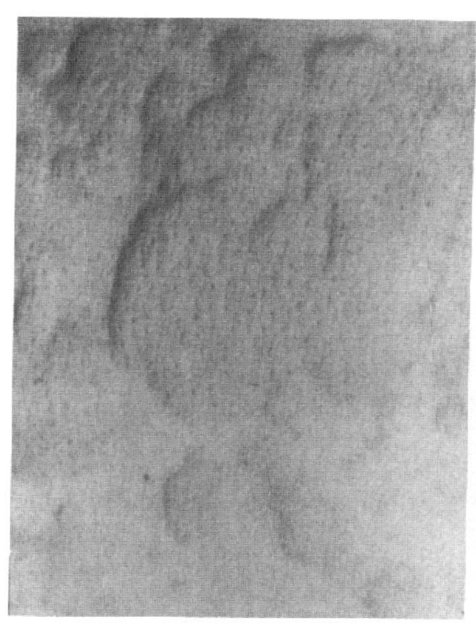

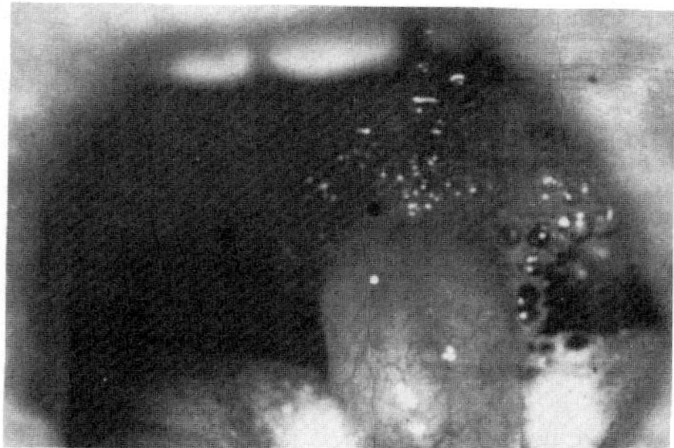

QUESTIONS:

1. What is the significance of this patient's symptoms and vital signs?
2. What is the pathophysiologic basis of this patient's signs and symptoms?
3. Is there any significance to the patient's past medical history?
4. Discuss the management and disposition of this patient.

ANSWERS:

1. Despite the fact that this patient has presented previously to the Emergency Department with chest pain, it is incumbent upon the emergency physician to rule out life-threatening disease. The constellation of symptoms of nasal stuffiness, feeling flushed, and chest tightness following an insect sting should suggest anaphylaxis. Anaphylaxis is the clinical syndrome characterized by the systemic reaction of various organ systems (usually the respiratory and dermatologic systems) to an antigen, in this case insect venom, causing an immunoglobulin E (IgE) mediated response. Apparently benign symptoms can rapidly progress to death within minutes.

Early in the course of anaphylaxis, the patient will often present with few or no objective findings and nonspecific symptoms such as itching, a lump in the throat, or a feeling of impending doom. This stage can rapidly progress to upper airway compromise secondary to edema, hypotension secondary to cardiovascular collapse, or severe bronchospasm. The degree of reaction varies greatly between patients.

Stings from the insect order Hymenoptera (bee, wasp, hornet, yellow jacket, fire ant) account for 50 to 80 deaths a year from allergy induced anaphylaxis. Only penicillin, accounting for 100 to 220 deaths a year, causes more anaphylactic deaths.

2. Anaphylaxis is a relatively immediate hypersensitivity reaction to an antigen such as an antibiotic, insect venom, food, or food additive. This results in the immunologic release or production of vasoactive mediators such as histamine, leukotrienes, and platelet activating factors. The syndrome of anaphylaxis comprises a broad range of signs and symptoms, ranging from mild pruritus to fatal cardiopulmonary collapse.

The venom of Hymenoptera insects is a mixture of proteins and peptides, all of which can induce the formation of IgE. This is considered the first stage, or sensitizing phase, of anaphylaxis. On subsequent reexposure, the already present antivenom IgE antibodies bind to mast cells and basophils, stimulating the release of histamine and related substances. These substances then promote smooth muscle spasm, increased vascular permeability, and peripheral vasodilation, resulting in cutaneous flushing, urticaria, angioedema, wheezing, and hypotension. It is interesting to note that half of the patients with insect sting related anaphylaxis cannot recall a prior sting.

3. There are two significant points in the patient's history that must be addressed. First is her history of mitral valve prolapse (MVP), also known as Barlow's syndrome. Mitral valve prolapse is characterized by an abnormal prolapse of one or both leaflets of the mitral valve into the left atrium during systole. It is reported to occur in 4 to 6% of females. Typically the patient with MVP is anxious and complains of chest pain or palpitations. These symptoms are often treated with beta blockers. While MVP could account for this patient's chest pain, it would not account for her other symptoms.

Of greater importance is the fact that the patient is on a beta blocker. Several authors have noted that patients on beta blockers who develop anaphylaxis have a more severe reaction and are more resistant to therapy. Speculation is that beta blockers inhibit adenylate cyclase, which causes a lowered level of intracellular cyclic AMP, and in turn leads to a lowered threshold for histamine and other anaphylactic mediator release. Also, beta blockers may facilitate bronchospasm and may cause a relative bradycardia inhibiting the cardiovascular response to hypotension.

Various modalities have been utilized to override the beta blocker effect, including atropine, isoproterenol, higher doses of epinephrine, and glucagon. Glucagon is thought to work by directly stimulating adenyl cyclase and increasing intracellular cyclic AMP, thus bypassing the beta receptor. The dose of glucagon is 5 to 10 mg given intravenously. Nausea, vomiting, hyperglycemia, and hypokalemia are the main side effects.

4. It is difficult to predict which patients demonstrating systemic signs and symptoms will go on to life-threatening anaphylaxis. Therefore, all patients with a suspected systemic reaction to an insect bite should be placed on a cardiac monitor, have intravenous access established, and be given supplemental oxygen. As most anaphylactic deaths are secondary to asphyxia due to laryngeal edema, bronchospasm, and mucous hypersecretion, the airway is the primary focus. It is always better to intubate early, as the anatomy can become rapidly distorted by impending angioedema. Vital signs must be monitored frequently, since a stable patient can rapidly deteriorate.

The goals of pharmacologic treatment are to try to reverse anaphylactic mediator release, reverse the effects of mediators already released, and block attachment of these mediators to end organs. In addition, local measures such as placing ice on the site of the sting may be effective. If the stinger is still present, it should be removed by flicking or scraping. Grasping with forceps can cause further release of venom from the sac.

Epinephrine is the cornerstone of treatment of anaphylaxis. Its beta effects help block the ongoing release of mediators from mast cells as well as cause smooth muscle relaxation and increase cardiac output. In addition, its alpha effects are beneficial in counteracting hypotension secondary to vasodilation. If the patient is relatively stable, 0.3 to 0.5 cc of 1:1000 epinephrine is administered subcutaneously at a site distant from the sting. This dose can be repeated in 20 minutes if necessary. In addition, there may be some efficacy to administering approximately 0.2 cc of 1:1000 epinephrine SC into the sting site to slow absorption.

If the patient has pronounced hypotension or impending airway compromise, epinephrine is administered intravenously. A 1:100,000 solution is utilized with 2 to 5 cc given as a slow bolus (some authors recommend an IV drip of 1 mg of epinephrine in 250 cc of D5W with titration to an adequate response). This dose can be repeated in 5 minutes. One final point is that age, the presence of ischemic heart disease, or presence of tachycardia are not considered absolute contraindications to the use of epinephrine. In these cases, the physician must simply be more diligent in monitoring the patient.

Antihistamines are also utilized to treat anaphylactic reactions, although in true anaphylaxis they are not first-line agents. Diphenhydramine, a histamine type 1 antagonist, can be administered at 1 to 2 mg/kg up to 50 mg, either intramuscularly or intravenously. Recent studies have advocated the use of histamine-2 blockers such as cimetidine given as a 300 mg bolus over 3 to 5 minutes.

While corticosteroids do not appear to play an immediate role, they do combat the late phase reactants. It is theorized that steroids stabilize membranes and inhibit the release of preformed granules in the mast cells. In addition, they block the effect of leukotrienes and chemotactic factors and reduce capillary leaking. Either methylprednisolone, as a 125 mg IV bolus, or hydrocortisone, as a 250 to 500 mg IV bolus, can be given.

As mentioned previously, the use of atropine, isoproterenol, and/or glucagon may be necessary for patients on beta blockers. Additionally, if bronchospasm is present, inhaled beta adrenergic agents (albuterol, metaproterenol) are useful as is aminophylline and ipratropium. Finally, in the patient with hypotension unresponsive to fluids (up to 3 L of Ringer's lactate may be necessary), dopamine, norepinephrine, and MAST garments may be necessary. Obviously, the more severe the degree of anaphylaxis, the greater the need for aggressive therapy.

Any patient with airway compromise, wheezing, or hypotension needs to be admitted for monitoring as do patients with a complicated history, namely the elderly, patients with a cardiac history, or patients on beta blockers. Patients who respond rapidly to minimal therapy such as one or two subcutaneous epinephrine injections can be discharged if they remain stable after 4 to 6 hours of observation. Discharge medications include diphenhydramine 25 to 50 mg every 6 hours for 3 days, and a 5-day tapering course of corticosteroids. Patients should be given explicit instructions to return if any symptoms recur. They should also follow up with their own physician in 24 hours. In addition, patients sensitive to bee venom should receive a prescription and instructions for either an Ana Kit or Epi Pen (these are bee sting kits containing epinephrine).

PEARLS:

1. In general, the shorter the duration between the sting and the onset of symptoms, the more severe the reaction.

2. Anaphylactic episodes tend to be more severe and are associated with greater morbidity and mortality in patients over 40 years of age.

3. If intravenous access cannot be obtained rapidly in the patient with life-threatening anaphylaxis, two other possible sites for rapid administration of epinephrine are via the endotracheal tube or injected sublingually into the rich venous network under the tongue.

4. Patients on beta blockers who develop anaphylactic shock unresponsive to epinephrine may respond to glucagon.

PITFALLS:

1. When removing the stinger of a honey bee, do not grasp it with forceps. This can result in further contraction of the venom sac. Instead, scrape from side to side.

2. Progression of symptoms is unpredictable. Any patient with systemic symptoms should have intravenous access established and be placed on a cardiac monitor.

3. Failure to intubate early in severe reactions can be a serious error. Progressive edema may cause distortion and friability of the normal laryngeal architecture. If severe distortion of airway anatomy is present, a surgical airway may be necessary.

4. Diphenhydramine does NOT reverse the effects of anaphylaxis. While it will block further binding of histamine, it does not antagonize histamine release or reverse the physiologic changes already induced by histamine binding.

5. Do not prematurely discharge a patient who has had a true anaphylactic reaction. These patients often relapse, particularly with bee stings where there may still be a depot of inciting antigen.

REFERENCES:

Jacobs RL, Rake GW, Fournier DC, et al. Potentiated anaphylaxis in patients with drug induced beta adrenergic blockade. J Allerg Clin Immunol 1987;68(2):125-127.

Mayumitt KS, Ascino M, et al. Intravenous cimetidine as an effective treatment for systemic anaphylaxis and acute allergic skin reaction. Ann Allerg 1987;58:447-451.

Settipane GA, Boyd GK. Anaphylaxis from insect stings: myths, controversy, and reality. Postgrad Med 1989;86:237-281.

Stafford CT: Life threatening allergic reactions: anticipating and preparing are the best defence. Postgrad Med 1989;86:235-245.

AN ELDERLY WOMAN WITH DIFFICULTY SPEAKING

Case 15:

A 67-year-old Hispanic female was brought in by her family, who stated she had had the sudden onset of drooling and difficulty speaking 1 hour earlier. The woman had been in he usual state of good health until that day, when she complained of a mild headache. While speaking with her daughter, she began to speak unintelligibly and drool profusely. Her daughter noted that her face appeared "twisted." The patient denied any history of diabetes, hypertension, heart disease, or stroke. She had never been hospitalized and in fact had not consulted a physician in over 40 years. Her family recalled one event which appeared somewhat similar to the current episode; approximately 2 years earlier, she had had a headache one day and lost consciousness, but regained consciousness spontaneously and refused to see a physician. Since that time, she had complained of frequent headaches. She was currently taking no medications and had no known allergies. Her family stated she had smoked a pack of cigarettes daily for the past 40 years. She drank no alcohol.

On examination, she was a plump elderly woman in no acute distress. Her blood pressure was 140/70, pulse was 82/minute and regular, respiratory rate 14/minute, and rectal temperature 98.8° F. Her head was atraumatic and normocephalic. Her extraocular movements were intact; conjunctivae anicteric; and the pupils were equal, round, and bilaterally reactive to light. Her optic fundi showed low-grade arteriovenous nicking, and the optic disk margins were sharp. Her neck was supple and her carotid arteries were 1+ bilaterally with normal upstrokes and no bruits. Her lungs had bibasilar crepitus posteriorly. Her heart sounds were normal, with no murmurs or gallops. Her abdomen was unremarkable. She had no edema of her extremities. Her neurologic exam revealed a left facial droop with some difficulty articulating words. Her family members stated that her speech had improved notably since the beginning of the episode. Her other cranial nerves were normal, her sensory and motor exam was unremarkable, and her gait and cerebellar exam were intact. Her deep tendon reflexes were 2+ and symmetrical; there were no Babinski's elicited.

DIAGNOSTIC CLUES:

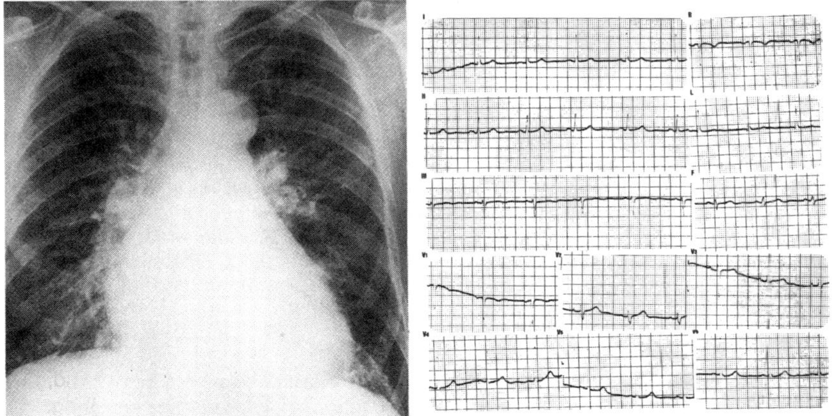

CAT scan of the head: Right posterior limb infarct

QUESTIONS:

1. What are the major syndromes of cerebrovascular ischemic disease?

2. Is the CAT scan of any help in making the diagnosis?

3. What further tests will need to be ordered in this patient?

4. Should this patient be anticoagulated?

5. What therapy should the patient receive?

ɔmes of cerebrovascular ischemic disease can be delineated

ɔcclusion due to atherogenic embolization or hypoperfusion
.tor artery occlusion due to atherosclerosis
ɔlization (typically ischemia in the distribution of a middle cerebral
ı or the distal posterior cerebral artery)
.l parenchyma hemorrhage, associated with hypertension,
ıy, or cerebral amyloid angiopathy
e. ,oid hemorrhage from an aneurysm or arteriovenous malformation

2. The CAT scan shows a small right posterior limb infarct, a lesion which is inconsistent with the patient's clinical presentation. It is probable that this lesion is old and that the current episode is either a transient ischemic attack (TIA) without a lesion or that the lesion is still too fresh to be imaged with the CAT scan. A CAT scan or MRI of the brain should be obtained in every patient with a TIA or stroke, in order to differentiate an infarct from a mass lesion, to determine if an infarct is bland or hemorrhagic, and to demonstrate the presence or absence of intracranial edema.

3. Although no bruits were auscultated, this patient's carotid pulses are diminished, and a carotid duplex is indicated. In the case of hemispheric symptoms or transient monocular blindness, a carotid duplex scan will reveal the presence or absence of a severe stenosis at the carotid bifurcation with over 90% sensitivity.

This patient's cardiogram is unremarkable. The EKG may show evidence of acute or chronic myocardial ischemia suggestive of mural thrombus formation as well as demonstrate any emboligenic arrhythmias. If the duplex scan is normal, a Holter monitor may demonstrate a sick sinus syndrome or transient arrhythmia. The patient's heart appears mildly enlarged. A two-dimensional echocardiogram may be useful to assess for a valvular disease, ventricular wall thrombus, or a hypokinetic area which might harbor thrombus.

Arteriography in older patients with hemispheric TIA or minor strokes should not be performed unless significant carotid bifurcation stenosis (greater than 70%) is suspected or demonstrated on carotid duplex. Patients undergoing arteriography should agree in advance to the possibility of carotid endarterectomy.

4. Heparin is indicated after a cardiac embolus, provided there are no systemic contraindications. Anticoagulation with heparin for patients with TIA or with stroke where more tissue is at risk distal to a large artery stenosis or recent occlusion may help prevent

thrombosis or distal propagation of thrombus, although there exists some controversy on this point. Heparin is absolutely contraindicated in hemispheric infarct accompanied by mass effect or in intracerebral hemorrhage. Continuous rather than bolus heparin therapy should be administered, with the goal of achieving a partial thromboplastin time of 1.5 times control.

Long-term anticoagulation is not without risk in the elderly. There exists an incidence of approximately 3 to 5% systemic complications and 2 to 4% cerebral hemorrhage yearly for elderly patients on chronic anticoagulation. Although arteriography carries a morbidity risk of under 3%, it may be warranted in order to clearly demonstrate a need for long-term anticoagulation.

5. Current therapy for a TIA aims to optimize cerebral blood flow and prevent thrombosis. In the event of stroke, the aim of therapy is to protect ischemic neurons and limit mass effect. Cardiac output should be maintained, particularly when ischemia is related to high-grade stenosis or occlusion. Support of cardiac output will help support collateral perfusion to ischemic areas. Except in subarachnoid hemorrhage, the systolic blood pressure need not be dropped below 170 initially. In the patient who threatens herniation due to intracerebral hemorrhage or large infarct, limitation of free water, diuretics such as furosemide, intravenous mannitol, and dexamethasone may help to prevent herniation. Aspirin remains the mainstay of medical therapy following a TIA or completed stoke. Randomized trials comparing surgical to medical treatment with aspirin in symptomatic patients with carotid stenosis need to be done. Until clear-cut recommendations are available, aspirin is generally preferable to endarterectomy where there is less than 70% carotid stenosis.

PEARLS:

1. Always attempt to localize the source of a patient's neurologic symptoms in the brain in order not to confuse peripheral with central lesions.

2. Be sure that the patient's current symptoms correspond anatomically with lesions found on CAT or MRI.

PITFALLS:

1. Never begin anticoagulation until intracerebral hemorrhage has been ruled out.

2. Elicit a detailed history before assuming that a patient is asymptomatic. Speak to the family or caretakers if necessary.

3. The absence of a bruit does not rule out carotid artery stenosis, as the bruit may disappear in high-grade stenosis.

REFERENCES:

Cerebral Embolism Task Force. Cardiogenic brain embolism. Arch Neurol 1986;43:71-76.

Dobkin BH. Management of geriatric TIA and stroke. Geriatrics 1988;43(11):27-34.

Meissner I, Wiebers D, Whisnant J, O'Fallon M. The natural history of asymptomatic carotid artery occlusive lesions. JAMA 1987;258:2704-2707.

Meyer F, Sundt T, et al. Focal cerebral ischemia: pathologic mechanisms and rationale for treatment. Mayo Clin Proc 1987;62:35-55.

SHOULDER PAIN FOLLOWING AN ELECTRIC SHOCK

Case 16:

A 65-year-old male presented to the Emergency Department complaining of pain in his right shoulder which began after he reached for an electrical wire lying in his backyard. He received an electric shock that lasted "for a few seconds" until he was able to release himself. His only complaint was nonradiating pain localized to the right shoulder. He denied chest pain, neck pain, shortness of breath, or abdominal pain. He stated he was previously in good health with a history of arthritis for which he occasionally required aspirin.

On physical examination, the patient was alert and cooperative but appeared in moderate discomfort. His vital signs revealed a blood pressure of 150/92, a regular pulse of 76/minute, and unlabored respirations at a rate of 16/minute. The skin was normal with no evidence of burns. Examination of the head, eyes, ears, nose, and throat was unremarkable. His neck was supple and there was no cervical spine tenderness on palpation. He had good breath sounds bilaterally, normal heart sounds, active bowel sounds, no abdominal tenderness, and a normal rectal examination.

The patient was holding his right arm internally rotated and close to the chest. The anterior aspect of the right shoulder appeared flat, with a more prominent coracoid process on the right compared to the left. He had normal pulses, good capillary refill, and no evidence of neurologic compromise in any of the extremities. The left arm and lower extremities had good active range of motion. An electrocardiogram as well as cervical spine and chest x-rays were interpreted as normal.

DIAGNOSTIC CLUE:

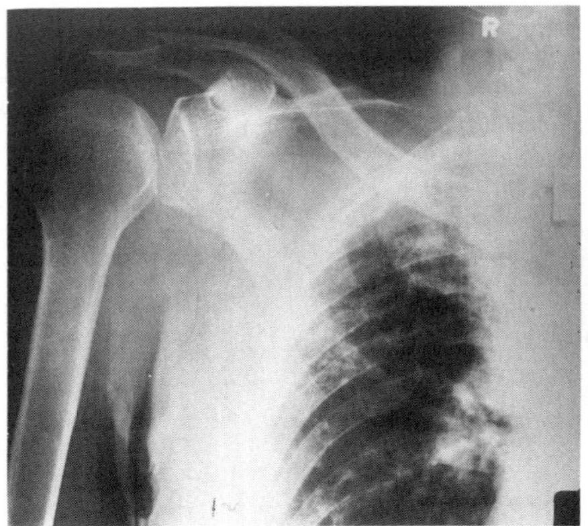

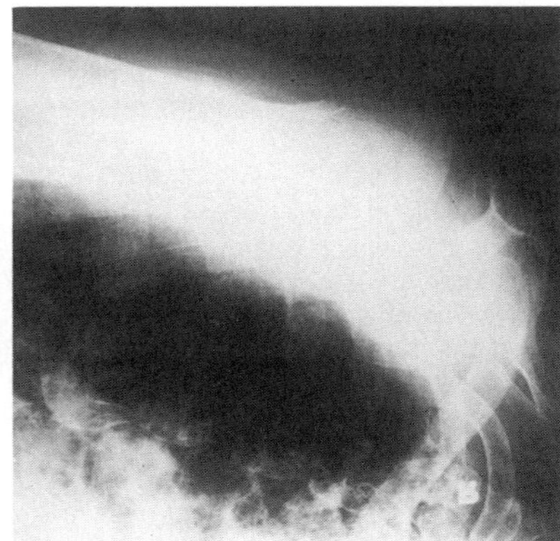

QUESTIONS:

1. What is the diagnosis?
2. What features help differentiate shoulder injuries?
3. What x-ray studies are most appropriate to adequately assess the shoulder joint?
4. What are the most common complications of this type of injury?

ANSWERS:

1. The diagnosis is posterior dislocation of the glenohumeral joint.

2. In a broad sense, the shoulder is thought to comprise the glenohumeral, acromioclavicular, and sternoclavicular joints. Of the three, the glenohumeral is the most precarious, having only soft restraints. Anterior dislocations account for over 95% of shoulder dislocations and are associated with an abduction, external rotation, and extension injury. The patient with an anterior dislocation usually presents supporting the dislocated arm or holding it to the side with the affected shoulder appearing squared-off with a prominent acromion process.

Posterior dislocations can be the result of a direct anterior-to-posterior blow, but are more commonly associated with an electric shock or convulsive seizure which causes the more powerful internal rotators to overpower the external rotators. The patient with a posterior dislocation presents with the affected arm held in adduction and internal rotation with the anterior aspect of the shoulder appearing flat with a prominent coracoid process. In addition, there may be a fullness around the scapula in a posterior dislocation.

The rarest of injuries to the glenohumeral joint is luxatoerecta dislocation. This is an inferior dislocation of the shoulder and is associated with severe hyperabduction. The patient presents with the arm held above the head 180 degrees elevated.

3. Whereas a routine AP shoulder film is often adequate to diagnose anterior dislocation, it is often inadequate to diagnose posterior dislocation. A true lateral (trans-scapular view) is the single best film for diagnosing posterior dislocation. A lateral x-ray shows the scapula as the letter Y: the vertical stem of the Y is projected by the body of the scapula and the upper fork of the Y is formed by the coracoid process and acromion process of the scapula. The glenoid fossa is located at the junction of the stem and two arms. In the normal shoulder, the humeral head is centered over this junction, while with posterior dislocations, the humeral head lies posterior to this junction. Conversely, with anterior dislocations the humeral head lies anterior to the junction.

4. Always document the neurovascular status of the involved arm prior to any reduction attempt. The axillary nerve and artery are particularly vulnerable with anterior dislocations in older patients. In addition, both anterior and posterior shoulder dislocations can have concomitant fractures (up to 50% in posterior dislocations). Luxatoerecta dislocations are always associated with rotator cuff tears.

The best method for reduction of dislocation is to achieve good relaxation using adequate analgesia and reassurance, and have the patient lie in the prone position with a 5- to 10-pound weight suspended from the wrist (not held in the hand).

PEARLS:

1. Blocking of external rotation and limitation of abduction is present in all cases of posterior dislocations of the shoulder.

2. Remember that even though posterior dislocations are relatively rare (approximately 3% of shoulder dislocations), they are often bilateral when present.

3. Subtle clues on the AP film may suggest a posterior dislocation: loss of the normal elliptical patten produced by overlap of the humeral head and posterior glenoid rim, or the humeral head appearing hollow or resembling a light bulb, or an isolated fracture of the lesser tuberosity.

4. Patients in whom radiographs of the shoulder are normal but whose presentation is similar to that of a dislocation may have suffered a dislocation that has spontaneously reduced, a subluxation, a rupture of the rotator cuff, an acromioclavicular joint injury, or an inapparent scapular fracture.

PITFALLS:

1. Posterior dislocations are the most commonly missed major dislocation, with 50% being overlooked.

2. The most common reasons for missing a posterior dislocation are failure to perform a careful examination and overreliance on x-rays which may be inadequate or misinterpreted.

3. While the great majority of shoulder pain is due to periarticular and articular disorders, the shoulder is also a common area for referred pain from the neck, great vessels, heart, lungs, mediastinum, diaphragm, and upper abdomen.

REFERENCES:

Bayley IJL, Kessel L. Posterior dislocation of the shoulder: the clinical spectrum. J Bone Joint Surg 1978;60B:440-448.

Butler ED, Gant TD. Electrical injuries with special reference to the upper extremities. Am J Surg 1977;134:95-101.

May VR. Posterior dislocation of the shoulder. Habitual, traumatic, and obstetrical. Orthop Clin North Am 1980;11:271-286.

Rockwood CA. Subluxations and dislocations about the shoulder. In: Rockwood CA, Green DP, eds. Fractures in adults 2nd ed. Philadelphia: JB Lippincott, 1984:722-860.

BURNS WITH A DIFFERENCE

Case 17:

A 17-year-old male was brought into the Emergency Department by police officers after he was found tampering with the "third rail" of a Mass Transit Authority train track. The patient complained of pain in his hands and right leg, and stated he might have "blacked out." His past medical history was unremarkable except for occasional insufflational use of cocaine (the patient denied recent use). He was unsure of his tetanus status.

His initial vital signs included a blood pressure of 150/90, a regular pulse of 76/minute, an unlabored respiratory rate of 24/minute, and a Glasgow Coma Scale score of 15. Initial inspection revealed second-degree burns of both palms, as well as second-degree with partial third-degree burns of the anterior neck, and third-degree burns of the right lower extremity (calf to foot circumferentially). Closer inspection also demonstrated blood around the right ear, no gross step-off fractures, and pupils approximately 3 mm in size, equal and reactive. The presence of priapism was noted. Examination of the chest, abdomen, and rectum was normal. The extremities demonstrated the aforementioned burns; in addition, there were exit burns on the plantar aspect of both feet. The dorsalis pedis and posterior tibial pulses were judged to be adequate bilaterally.

DIAGNOSTIC CLUES:

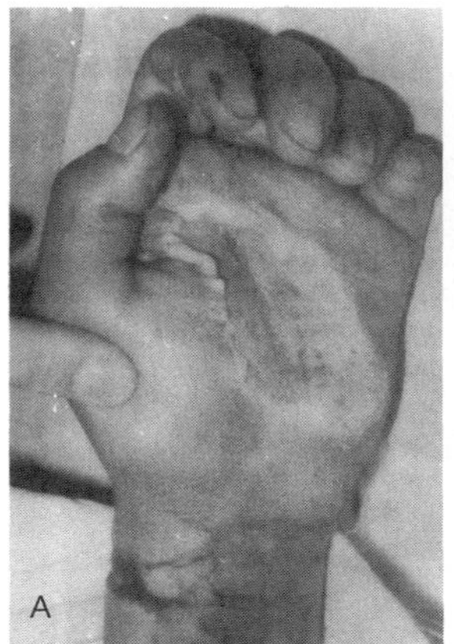
A

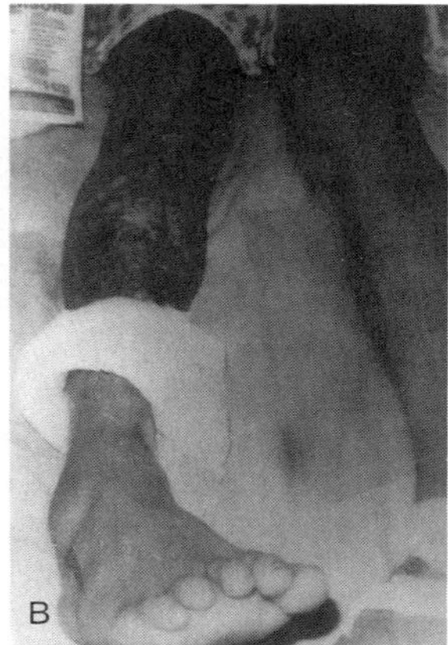
B

QUESTIONS:

1. What factors influence an electrical injury?
2. What are the various "types" of electrical injury?
3. What are the early clinical manifestations of an electrical injury?
4. What are the late manifestations of an electrical injury?
5. What is the appropriate management for this patient?

ANSWERS:

1. There are many factors which influence the severity of electrical injuries. Much of this is centered around Ohm's law, which states that I = V/R, in which the amperage (I), or amount of current flow per unit time, is equal to the voltage (V), the difference of electrical potential between two points, divided by the resistance (R), which is the opposition to current flow.

Other factors to be aware of include the type of current (alternating versus direct), the current pathway, duration of contact, and surface area of contact. Generally speaking, alternating currents are felt to be more damaging than direct currents because the tetanizing effect of alternating current prolongs contact time.

In addition, the relative resistance of various tissues determines the path of current flow, with bone having the highest resistance and blood and nerve vessels the lowest. Skin resistance varies with its relative moisture content, with dry skin having a resistance of approximately 1,000,000 Ohms and wet skin only 300 Ohms.

2. There are several types of electrical injury. These include direct electrical injury, which involves the passage of current through the skin and usually exhibits entrance and exit wounds; arc burns, which occur when the current is external to the body where the depth of the burn will be determined by the proximity of the current to the skin; and flame burns, which are thermal injuries resulting form a direct flame or ignition of clothing, resulting in essentially a thermal burn.

3. Early manifestations of electrical injury include cardiac arrest (both ventricular fibrillation and asystole), respiratory arrest, hypertension, seizures, mental status changes, paresis/paralysis, myoglobinuria and renal failure, fractures and dislocations involving both the spine and extremities, gastrointestinal symptoms, and vascular thrombosis and hemorrhage.

4. Delayed clinical manifestations include ascending paresis, transverse myelitis, incomplete spinal cord transection, cataracts, and hemorrhage.

5. Initial management in this patient is the same as in all severely injured patients, i.e., assessing the airway, ventilation and circulatory status with an emphasis on spinal immobilization (particularly in light of the patient's possible loss of consciousness).

While the patient is being disrobed, pay special attention to location of entrance and exit wounds. The patient should be placed on a cardiac monitor, and at least two large bore intravenous catheters should be inserted. A nasogastric tube should be placed to decompress the stomach as well as to check for gastric bleeding, and bladder catheterization should be performed to assist in fluid management and to check for myoglobinuria.

Initial fluid therapy consists of aggressive administration of isotonic crystalloids, with the goal of maintaining a urine output of 1 to 2 cc/kg/hour. In addition, if myoglobinuria is present, attempts should be made to alkalinize the urine at least to blood pH, and early use of osmotic agents such as mannitol (approximately 25 g initially) should be considered.

Therapy for cardiac and neurologic dysfunction should be based on standard guidelines. Blood studies should include CBC, arterial blood gases, electrolytes, BUN, and creatinine with frequent reassessment based on the clinical picture. In addition, the patient should be typed and crossed for at least four units of packed red blood cells. Early collaboration with a surgeon is necessary in order to determine the need for debridement and exploration of wounds.

PEARLS:

1. Early aggressive management with large fluid volumes, alkalinization of the urine, and osmotic diuretics will help limit complications.

2. The presence of pain and tenderness over the shoulder and scapular regions should raise the suspicion of posterior shoulder dislocation (often associated with electrical injuries).

3. Respect gastrointestinal symptoms. These can be a warning of serious complications, including intestinal perforation.

4. Follow the hematocrit closely.

5. Explore full-thickness injuries early rather than late.

6. Ventricular fibrillation is associated with alternating current, while asystole is seen with direct current injuries (particularly lightning strikes, which are high-voltage, direct current injuries).

PITFALLS:

1. Do not hesitate to refer the patient to a specialty center. Electrical injuries may be deceiving. Extensive tissue destruction may be present despite relatively innocuous burns.

Electricity can cause thrombosis of any vessel leading to delayed tissue or organ destruction.

2. Do not rely on burn formulas to estimate fluid requirements since much of the injury is hidden.

3. Be sure to order necessary x-rays to help diagnose fractures and dislocations.

4. Have the patient examined by an ophthalmologist for cataract formation, which can occur up to 1 year later.

REFERENCES:

Comer RW, Fitchie, JG, Caughman WF, Zwemer JD. Oral trauma. Emergency care of lacerations, fractures, and burns. Postgrad Med 1989;85(2):34-37.

Epperly TD, Stewart JR. The physical effects of lightning injury. J Fam Pract 1989;29(3):267-272.

Hammond JS, Ward CG. High-voltage electrical injuries: management and ouctome of 60 cases. South Med J 1988;81(11):1351-1352.

Purdue GF, Hunt JL. Inhalation injuries and burns in the inner city. Surg Clin North Am 1991;71(2):385-397.

A STAB WOUND TO THE NECK

Case 18:

A 19-year-old male walked into the Emergency Department stating that he had been stabbed in the neck approximately 30 minutes earlier. The patient's vital signs were stable. On examination, a single 1½-inch laceration was seen just anterior to the midportion of the right sternocleidomastoid muscle with violation of the platysma. There were no other significant findings on examination.

DIAGNOSTIC CLUE:

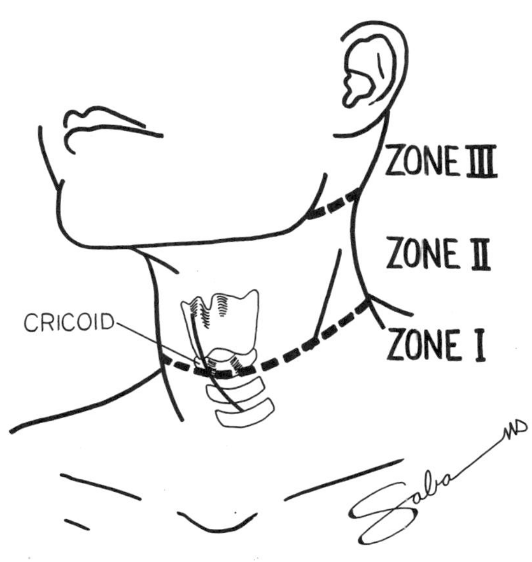

QUESTIONS:

1. What are the immediate concerns in the management of a patient with a penetrating neck injury?

2. What structures are at greatest risk for injury and what are the clinical manifestations of injury to each?

3. Which group of patients requires immediate surgery?

4. Describe the major landmarks of the neck used to determine the treatment plan.

ANSWERS:

1. As with all trauma victims, the initial approach to a patient with a penetrating neck would should begin with the ABC's—that is, rapid assessment and control of the airway, breathing, and circulation—and cervical spine stabilization if indicated.

It may be necessary to intubate the patient if spontaneous respirations are inadequate, blood or vomitus cannot be cleared, or progressive swelling threatens to occlude the airway. However, there are attendant risks in intubating a patient with neck trauma; one may induce the patient to gag or cough, potentially dislodging a clot and provoking massive bleeding from an injured vessel. In addition, the anatomy may become so distorted that oral intubation is impossible. It is for this reason that the physician managing a patient with a penetrating neck wound must be prepared to perform a cricothyroidotomy. However, despite this risk of exacerbating bleeding, maintenance of the airway takes precedence over risk of hemorrhage.

The physician must also ensure adequate breathing in a patient with a penetrating wound to the neck. Bear in mind that penetrating injuries, particularly at the base of the neck , may violate the chest cavity and puncture the lung with a resulting pneumothorax and/or hemothorax.

Bleeding in the neck can usually be controlled by direct pressure, although injuries at the base of the neck and high up in the neck may be more difficult to control. At the same time that hemorrhage is controlled, intravenous access should be obtained with at least two large-bore catheters (14G or 16G). If the possibility exists of injury to the innominate or subclavian vein, one of the intravenous catheters should be placed in a lower extremity and the other in the upper extremity on the uninjured side.

The initial assessment should also include careful examination for disability. It is important to remember that not only is the spinal cord susceptible but so are the phrenic, recurrent laryngeal, and cranial nerves as well as the brachial plexus. The presence of a neurologic deficit may also signal an injury to the carotid or vertebral artery with resultant central nervous system ischemia.

A final point is the need to ensure that the patient's entire body is exposed and examined, inasmuch as injury to other areas of the body may be missed if attention is drawn entirely to an obvious stab wound of the neck. After completion of all of the above, a cervical x-ray and a chest x-ray should be obtained as well as the proper blood specimens ordered, including a complete blood count and type and cross-match.

2. The reasons injuries to the neck are so potentially dangerous is because of the large number of anatomically important structures confined to a relatively small space. In addition, life-threatening injuries in the neck do not always present in an obvious way

immediately and can easily be overlooked. It is for this reason that the physician caring for a patient with a neck wound must be well-versed in the presentations of injuries to this area.

Injury	Significant Findings
Carotid artery	Coma, focal neurologic findings, hematoma (frequently expanding), hemorrhage, hypotension, pulse deficit, thrill or bruit
Jugular vein	Hematoma, hemorrhage, hypotension
Larynx and trachea	Hoarseness, stridor, dysphagia, dysphonia, hemoptysis, subcutaneous emphysema, flattening of the anterior neck
Esophagus	Dysphagia, drooling, subcutaneous emphysema, bloody nasogastric aspirate,* air in the prevertebral space on lateral cervical x-ray

*Do not insert nasogastric tube if injury to the base of the neck is present.

3. Immediate surgical exploration of a penetrating wound to the neck is indicated if there is any evidence of active bleeding, an expanding hematoma, hypovolemic shock, respiratory distress, hoarseness, subcutaneous emphysema, blood in the aerodigestive tract, or a neurologic deficit.

4. After stabilization, the first step in evaluating the wound to the neck is to determine if the platysma has been violated. In this regard, the platysma is treated much like the peritoneum of the abdomen—if it is violated, surgical consultation is mandatory. The neck can also be viewed as anterior and posterior triangles, with the sternocleidomastoid muscle serving as the demarcation. Most of the major vascular and visceral structures are in the anterior triangle portion. Zones of the neck are described for determining treatment plan (see diagram on page 91).

Zone I	Base of the neck to the cricoid cartilage level
Zone II	Between the angle of the mandible and cricoid cartilage
Zone III	Above the angle of the mandible

Zone II injuries are the most common, while Zone I and Zone III injuries usually require arteriography to help determine if surgery is indicated.

PEARLS:

1. Physical findings in a neck wound may be deceptive in that an apparently small hematoma may conceal a much larger, deeply confined subfascial collection of blood.

2. If there is difficulty in resuscitating a patient with a neck wound, be sure to consider the possibility of intrathoracic injury, i.e., massive hemothorax and/or tension pneumothorax.

3. If there is a suspected jugular venous injury, the patient's head should be kept lower than the heart to diminish the chance of air embolization.

4. In any patient with positive neurologic findings, be suspicious of carotid or vertebral artery injury as well as nerve damage.

PITFALLS:

1. Do not force the endotracheal tube when intubating, as this may complete a partial transection or cause a completely transected trachea to migrate into the mediastinum.

2. Do not remove an embedded object in the Emergency Department, since it may be tamponading a hemorrhage.

3. Do not probe wounds in the Emergency Department, since this action may dislodge a clot resulting in a massive hemothorax or create an iatrogenic pneumothorax.

4. Do not clamp vessels. Apply direct pressure instead.

REFERENCES:

Carducci B, Lowe RA, Dalsey W. Collective review: penetrating neck trauma: consensus and controversies. Ann Emerg Med 1986;15:208-215.

Jurkovich GJ, Zingarelli W, Wallace J et al. Penetrating neck trauma: diagnostic studies in the asymptomatic patient. J Trauma 1985;23:819-822.

McInnis WD, Cruz AB, Aust JB, et al. Penetrating injuries to the neck: pitfalls in the management. Am J Surg 1975;130:416-420.

Merion RM, Harness JK, Ramsberg SR, et al. Selective management of penetrating neck trauma: cost implications. Arch Surg 1981;116:691-696.

Narrod JA, Moore EE. Initial management of penetrating neck wounds: a selective approach. J Emerg Med 1984;2:17-22.

Rao PM, Bhatti MF, Gaudino J, et al. Penetrating injuries to the neck: criteria for exploration. J Trauma 1983;23:47-49.

LOW BACK PAIN

Case 19:

A 34-year-old male was brought to the Emergency Department by paramedics after being found unconscious in the street. The patient admitted to intravenous cocaine and heroin use as well as drinking large quantities of wine. He complained of low back pain, which he stated had been present for several weeks but had worsened over the past few days. He added that he had been seen in another Emergency Department 2 weeks ago, where x-rays were found to be normal and he was prescribed bedrest and ibuprofen. The patient stated he had been dissatisfied with this therapy and needed "something strong" for pain relief.

Physical examination showed a lethargic but arousable male with an oral temperature of 99.4° F, pulse of 94/minute and regular, blood pressure of 108/76, and respiratory rate of 20/minute. Numerous track marks were noted on his upper extremities, but there were no skin abscesses. The neck was supple without lymphadenopathy. The chest was clear, and there were no heart murmurs auscultated. The abdomen was soft with decreased bowel sounds. The patient stated he was unable to stand because of pain. There was tenderness to palpation over the lower lumbar spinous processes. Straight leg raising was limited to 45 degrees bilaterally, with the patient complaining of pain radiating down the right leg. There was decreased sensation to pinprick over the S1 dermatome of the right leg. The other sensory modalities, strength, stretch reflexes, and rectal tone were normal. A complete blood count and lumbosacral x-rays were interpreted as normal.

DIAGNOSTIC CLUE:

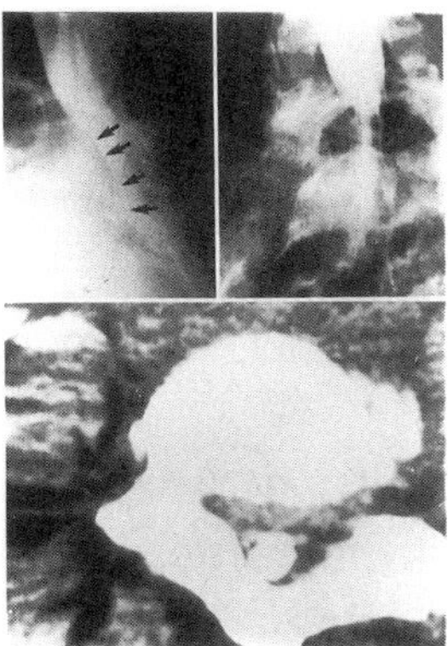

QUESTIONS:

1. Based on the history and physical examination, what is the differential diagnosis?

2. What are the warning symptoms of "dangerous" low back pain?

3. Which ancillary tests help establish the diagnosis?

4. What is the indicated treatment for this patient?

ANSWERS:

1. Because of its prevalence, it is easy to dismiss the patient with low back pain, particularly the intravenous drug abuser who is often viewed as a "drug seeker." However, it is the important task of the Emergency Department physician to rule out serious disease rather than merely confirm the diagnosis of lumbar strain or sprain.

In this patient, the possible etiologies of low back pain are limitless, but the first concern must be elimination of life-threatening causes of back pain. The physician must consider meningitis, bacterial endocarditis (in one study 25% of patients with bacterial endocarditis had low back pain as the predominant complaint), vertebral osteomyelitis (bacterial, tuberculous, fungal), transverse myelitis, lymphoma (HIV-related), and epidural abscess as well as referred pain (pyelonephritis, pancreatitis, splenic abscess, etc.).

2. While the history may be loaded with pitfalls and often patients believe they must amplify their complaints in order to obtain adequate pain relief, certain clues may serve as warning signals for serious disease. Be suspicious of unrelenting progressive pain, pain unrelieved by bedrest, fever or chills, history of parenteral drug abuse, alcoholism, corticosteroid use, anticoagulant therapy, immunocompromise, history of cancer, or a change in bowel or bladder function.

3. Routine laboratory tests can be woefully misleading in the evaluation of low back pain. Often the white blood cell count and routine radiographs are normal even with life-threatening conditions. It is of interest that the erythrocyte sedimentation rate has been found to be elevated in 90% of patients with an epidural abscess. A urinalysis can also be a valuable screening test. If meningitis is strongly suspected, a spinal tap is indicated, although this should be performed with caution because the spinal tap may drain an abscess cavity, precipitating intradural spread of the infection.

The myelogram is the most sensitive radiographic evaluation for spinal epidural abscess. Computerized tomography can add information by demonstrating epidural compression or revealing a continuous paraspinal abscess. Bone scans can also be helpful in detecting early infection when plain films appear normal. As more experience is accumulated with MRI, this modality offers promise in supplanting the myelogram as the diagnostic procedure of choice in diagnosing spinal cord compression.

4. The most important factor in successful treatment of spinal epidural abscess is early identification. The problem lies in the fact that the early presentation of spinal epidural abscess is nonspecific, i.e., localized pain and tenderness. Once a neurologic deficit occurs, the prognosis for full recovery worsens. In the intravenous drug abuser, antibiotic therapy should be directed to Gram-negative organisms as well as *Staphylococcus*

aureus, pending culture results. When neurologic deficits are present, or the patient appears toxic, emergent decompressive laminectomy is indicated.

PEARLS:

1. The clinician must consider spinal epidural abscess in any patient with back pain who is immunocompromised, an intravenous drug abuser, has had previous spinal surgery, is an alcoholic, or has had a recent urinary tract infection or manipulation.

2. The progression of symptoms of spinal epidural abscess is highly variable, often initially presenting as only localized pain or a patient who refuses to walk.

3. While Staphylococcus aureus accounts for the vast majority of cases of spinal epidural abscess in the normal host, in intravenous drug abusers the physician must also consider Gram-negative organisms as well as Mycobacterium tuberculosis.

4. Be sure to inquire about any change in bowel or bladder function in any patient with low back pain.

5. Back pain that does not improve with bedrest is always worrisome.

6. True muscle weakness is the most reliable indicator of continuing loss of nerve conduction. Sensory changes are subjective and reflexes lost in a previous episode of nerve root compression rarely return.

PITFALLS:

1. The most common mistake is failure to consider the diagnosis of spinal epidural abscess. It is easy to disregard the patient with low back pain, but it is important to remember that pain induces anxiety more often than anxiety induces pain.

2. Both the white blood cell count and temperature can be normal in spinal epidural abscess.

3. Spine roentgenograms are misleading since it takes several weeks for effects of osteomyelitis to appear on plain x-ray. Conversely, early changes such as narrowed disk spaces are often attributed to degenerative disk disease rather than infection.

4. Another common error is failure to document rectal tone. In all but the most straightforward cases, the clinician should perform a rectal exam, checking for rectal tone, prostatic consistency, occult blood in the stool, and most important, sensation in the rectal

area, which is innervated by S2, S3, and S4. Absence of sensation in this area suggests central lumbar compression, a neurosurgical emergency.

5. Also make sure an accurate temperature is recorded. In patients who are tachypneic or mouth breathers, this must be a rectal temperature.

REFERENCES:

Baker AS, Ojemann RC, Swartz MN, et al. Spinal epidural abscess. N Engl J Med 1975;293:463-468.

Churchill MA, Geraci JE, Hunder GG. Musculoskeletal manifestations of bacterial endocarditis. Ann Int Med 1977;87:754-759.

Danner RL, Hartman BJ. Update of spinal epidural abscesses: 35 cases and review of the literature. Rev Infect Dis 1987;9:265-274.

Koppel BS, Tuchman AJ, Mangiardi JR, et al. Epidural spine infection in intravenous drug abusers. Arch Neurol 1988;45:1331-1337.

Levy DB, Borenstein M. Emergency department management of low back pain. Topics Emerg Med 1989;11:11-28.

A SENIOR CITIZEN WITH ABDOMINAL PAIN

Case 20:

A 77-year-old white male was referred to the Emergency Department by his private physician because of progressive abdominal discomfort for 2 weeks. He was a healthy and active senior citizen whose past medical history was significant only for mild hypertension controlled with a low-salt diet. Approximately 2 weeks earlier, he noted the onset of profuse diarrhea with malaise and abdominal discomfort. His stool was brown and watery without any melena or frank blood, and he reported up to six bowel movements daily. He consulted his private physician, who advised bedrest and fluids. His stool was guaiac negative at that time and a stool culture was reported as negative 3 days later.

The diarrhea persisted, accompanied by diffuse abdominal discomfort and mild cramping. The patient noted some small improvement in the consistency of the stool with the use of over-the-counter antidiarrheal preparations. He consulted his physician again 1 week later, at which time he was found to be afebrile and well-hydrated. His abdomen was not tender, and there was no visceromegaly or masses. His bowel sounds were very active. Rectal exam was unremarkable and his stool was guaiac negative. A stool sample sent for ova and parasites was reported as negative 3 days later.

The patient noted persistent abdominal discomfort, frequent stools, and progressive malaise over the following week. He returned once again to his physician, who found him to have a fever of 100.2° F rectally and mild abdominal distention; the physician referred him to the Emergency Department for further evaluation.

In the Emergency Department, the patient was a well-nourished, well-developed white male who appeared younger than his stated age. He appeared to be in moderate discomfort, complaining of diffuse abdominal discomfort. His blood pressure was 150/88, his pulse was 90/minute and regular, his respiratory rate was 16/minute, and a rectal temperature was 100.4° F. His lungs were clear, and his cardiac examination was normal. His abdomen was slightly distended with mild diffuse tenderness. His liver and spleen were normal in size and consistency. There was no ascites and no palpable masses. His bowel sounds were hyperactive. Stool was trace guaiac positive.

DIAGNOSTIC CLUES:

Serum white blood cell count: 17,100
Differential count: 84 polymorphonuclear leukocytes, 6 bands, and 10 lymphocytes
Hematocrit: 44%
Mean corpuscular volume: 86
Platelet count: 222,000

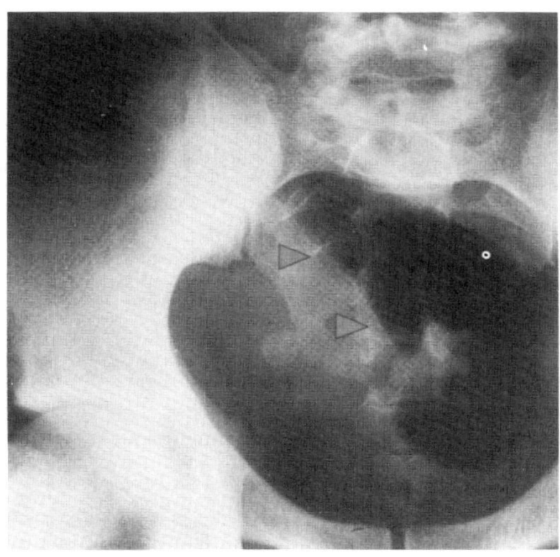

QUESTIONS:

1. What is the differential diagnosis of this patient's abdominal discomfort?

2. What factors must be taken into consideration in evaluating the elderly patient with an acute intraabdominal process?

3. What is the significant finding on x-ray?

4. Should any further diagnostic procedure be performed at this point?

5. What are possible sequelae for this patient if the correct diagnosis is overlooked?

ANSWERS:

1. The diagnosis of acute abdominal disease in the elderly is often very difficult. Possibilities to be considered in this case include infectious causes of diarrhea, intestinal parasites, intestinal obstruction, appendicitis, diverticulitis, and colonic volvulus. Less common possibilities include such systemic disorders as Addison's disease and porphyria.

A serious problem in the elderly is incarceration or strangulation of an asymptomatic external hernia. These account for nearly 30% of acute intestinal obstructions, with a mortality rate of 44% associated with emergency surgical intervention.

Elderly patients with systemic illnesses and poor mobility may develop massive gaseous distention of the large bowel even in the absence of actual mechanical obstruction. This form of colonic pseudoobstruction, known as Ogilvie's syndrome, can be decompressed effectively via colonoscopy, avoiding the risks of surgery.

2. Elderly patients with abdominal pain present a diagnostic challenge. The history, so critical in the evaluation of the acute abdomen, may be difficult to obtain in the patient who has suffered cognitive decline. Associated degenerative or disease processes may suppress classic physical findings. Tenderness, pain, muscle rigidity, and guarding may be diminished or absent. The febrile response may be blunted or absent, and leukocytosis generally does not occur to the same degree as in the younger patient. The picture is further complicated by the fact that multiple abdominal disorders may coexist and lead to diagnostic confusion.

Elderly patients tend to delay in seeking medical care, and a significant percentage will present more than 48 hours after onset of symptoms. Contributing factors may include reluctance to seek assistance, social isolation, economic factors, dislike of hospitalization, fear of death, and altered perception of symptoms.

Significant differences in pathophysiology exist between old and young patients. The appendix in older patients is frequently atrophic with decreased lymphatic tissue and a narrowed or obliterated lumen. Mucosal thinning, fatty infiltration, and fibrosis of the wall are commonly seen. The appendiceal blood supply is decreased due to associated vascular disease. All of these factors contribute to a more rapid progression of appendicitis in the older patient and an increased incidence of perforation.

3. This patient's abdominal x-ray reveals an appendicolith. Plain abdominal films may show an appendicolith in 7 to 12% of patients with right lower quadrant pain. When present, an appendicolith is nearly always associated with appendicitis.

4. Barium enema has been advocated for further evaluation of suspected appendicitis in children as well as adults. The barium enema in appendicitis reveals nonfilling or only partial filling of the appendix, a mass effect on the cecum from the inflamed appendix, or rigidity of the cecum. Unfortunately, barium enema may result in a relatively high incidence of false-negative and false-positive readings in appendicitis.

Recently, the medical literature has contained a number of reports of the use of high-resolution real-time ultrasonography with abdominal compression for the diagnosis of appendicitis. However, the data do not yet indicate greater accuracy in diagnosis compared to clinical judgment alone.

Laparoscopy may be of value in the evaluation of the patient with equivocal findings, such as a child with an unclear clinical presentation or a woman of childbearing age with right lower quadrant pain. When used in highly selected groups, laparoscopy has prevented laparotomy in up to one-third of patients. However, laparoscopy is often performed under general anesthesia, and patients are not spared an invasive procedure. A recent development is appendectomy performed via laparoscope, with reduction in healing time for the surgical wound.

5. The most significant risk is that of appendiceal perforation, an event which carries with it a mortality rate of 25% in patients over age 75. When symptoms have persisted for more than 48 hours, the risk of perforation is quite high. Once tissue necrosis and perforation occur, the risk of complications is greatly increased. Possible complications include abscess formation, peritonitis, sepsis, small bowel obstruction, pyogenic abscess of the liver, and enterocutaneous fistula.

PEARLS:

1. Although clinical criteria are paramount in making the diagnosis of acute appendicitis, the presentation can be atypical in as many as 45% of patients.

2. An "unnecessary" operation is preferable to an unnecessary perforation.

PITFALLS:

1. Although appendicitis is less common in the elderly than in the young, its severity is much greater. Over 50% of deaths associated with appendicitis occur in the elderly.

2. A short period of observation in the Emergency Department or hospital may be helpful, but prolonged observation will change the possibility of perforation into a certainty.

REFERENCES:

Horattas MC, Guyton DP, Wu D. A reappraisal of appendicitis in the elderly. Am J Surg 1990;160(3):291-293.

Irvin TT. Abdominal pain: a surgical audit of 1190 emergency admissions. Br J Surg 1989;76(11):1121-1125.

Klein SR, Layden L, Wright JF, White RA. Appendicitis in the elderly. A diagnostic challenge. Postgrad Med 1988;83(8):247-254.

Phillips SL, Burns GP: Acute abdominal disease in the aged. Med Clin North Am 1988;72(5):1213-1224.

Poole GV: Appendicitis. The diagnostic challenge continues. Am Surg 1988;54(10):609-612.

TESTICULAR PAIN IN A YOUNG MAN

Case 21:

A 20-year-old black male was brought to the Emergency Department by his college basketball coach because the student was complaining of acute testicular pain for 1 hour. The patient was a healthy, athletic student with no prior medical history. During a practice session, several players had collided and the patient was found on the floor clutching his genitals in great pain. The pain was most severe over the left testicle, but radiated into the abdominal and inguinal regions bilaterally. The patient was not certain if he had suffered direct testicular trauma during the collision. The patient stated he had noted intermittent left testicular pain over the past several weeks, with episodes lasting up to 10 minutes but resolving spontaneously. He denied any urethral discharge or frequency. He was sexually active without any history of venereal infection.

On physical examination, the patient was found to be in acute distress, diaphoretic and groaning in pain. Blood pressure was 140/90, pulse was 120/minute and regular, respiratory rate was 20/minute and regular, and rectal temperature was 99.1° F. His scrotum appeared erythematous with slight edema of the scrotal skin. The left testicle was exquisitely tender to palpation but appeared to be in normal position. Elevation and support of the testis did not relieve the pain. There was no penile discharge and no inguinal adenopathy. Rectal exam revealed a nontender prostate of normal consistency.

DIAGNOSTIC CLUES:

Urinalysis:

Specific gravity	1.010
pH	5
WBC	0-2/hpf
RBC	0-2/hpf
Casts	None seen
Bacteria	None seen
Crystals	None seen

QUESTIONS:

1. What are the diagnostic possibilities in this patient?

2. What is the pathogenesis of this condition?

3. What aspects of this patient's presentation are atypical?

4. Should any further diagnostic tests be performed?

5. What treatment could be initiated in the Emergency Department?

ANSWERS:

1. The most likely diagnosis is testicular torsion, given the acute presentation following trauma and the absence of any urethral symptomatology. However, the diagnosis of acute scrotal pain in a young man may be difficult, due to the rising number of cases of epididymitis. As a general rule, however, a young man with an acutely painful scrotum, irritative voiding symptoms, urethral discharge, and pyuria probably has epididymitis rather than testicular torsion.

2. Two factors appear to be responsible for testicular torsion. The first is a congenital anomaly which enables the spermatic cord to twist. If the tunica vaginalis surrounds the epididymis as well as the testis, the testis is prevented from creating its normal strong attachment to the scrotal wall (the bell clapper deformity). Another possible anomaly is incomplete attachment of the testis to the epididymis, allowing the testis to twist around an elongated mesorchium.

The second factor is a force that rotates the testis and holds it in that position. A strong contraction of the cremaster muscle can rotate the testis. Common precipitating events include strenuous exercise, sexual activity, or trauma.

The type and extent of testicular damage depend on the degree of torsion and its duration. Experimental reports have indicated that 360 degrees of torsion causes cellular necrosis within 12 to 24 hours, whereas three complete turns cause necrosis within 2 hours.

The primary pathologic features of torsion are ischemia and impeded venous and lymphatic drainage. The Sertoli and germ cells are the first to be affected. Death of the Leydig cells follows somewhat later. Long-term sequelae include testicular atrophy as well as abnormalities in the structure, number, motility, and viability of sperm and altered serum concentrations of LH and FSH.

3. The patient is somewhat old for presentation with testicular torsion. As a general rule, testicular torsion is a disorder of children and teenagers. It is uncommon over age 30, but should nonetheless be considered in the differential diagnosis of scrotal pain in patients of all ages.

The patient's history of intermittent testicular pain is not atypical. Some studies have indicated that over 35% of patients report prior similar episodes of pain, which are presumably episodes of torsion with spontaneous resolution.

4. When diagnosis cannot be made from the history or clinical picture, an attempt may be made perform Doppler studies of the spermatic arteries in the ED and compare both

sides. Two additional useful studies are Doppler ultrasound and radionuclide scanning. False-positive and false-negative results are uncommon with both of these tests. Unfortunately, these tests are often not available on an emergency basis when a patient presents with acute torsion. In addition, many authors argue that every minute wasted in diagnosis results in further testicular compromise.

5. If a patient presents with a case of possible torsion and no urologist or general surgeon will be available for several hours, an attempt at manual detorsion is indicated. Sedation may be given before detorsion is attempted; however, some authors prefer no anesthesia and are guided by the patient's response after each step. With torsion, the right testis twists clockwise and the left testis twists counterclockwise.

For manual detorsion, the physician should pronate his or her hand, take hold of the affected testicle gently but securely, and rotate it by supination 180 degrees. If the pain is alleviated, the physician can continue in 180 degree increments until the pain is relieved. If the pain is worsened, the procedure should be repeated in the opposite direction.

Even if manual detorsion is successful, it is absolutely necessary for the patient to undergo bilateral orchiopexy as soon as possible, to prevent recurrence and possible future testicular damage.

PEARLS:

1. Since testicular torsion is not common, entertainment of the diagnosis must be based on suspicion, not experience.

2. Even a fully documented history of prior orchiopexy does not provide assurance that the testicle has not torsed again.

3. The sooner a torsion is relieved, the better the end result will be.

PITFALLS:

1. Testicular torsion is a urologic emergency in which every minute counts. Do not delay treatment in order to obtain further diagnostic information.

2. The Prehn sign (in which elevation and support of the testis relieves the pain of epididymitis and orchitis but not that of torsion) is not infallible. The physician must rely on clinical judgment.

REFERENCES:

Cass AS. Torsion of the testis. Postgrad Med 1990;87(1):69-70, 73-74.

Jones DJ, Macreadie D, Morgans BT. Testicular torsion in the armed services; twelve year review of 179 cases. Br J Surg 1986;73(8):624-626.

Lindsey D, Stanisic TH. Diagnosis and management of testicular torsion: pitfalls and perils. Am J Emerg Med 1988;6(1):42-46.

Sheldon CA. Undescended testis and testicular torsion. Surg Clin North Am 1985;65(5):1303-1329.

Young GP. Abdominal catastrophes. Emerg Med Clin North Am 1989;7(3):699-720.

EPISTAXIS

Case 22:

A 65-year-old hypertensive male presented to the Emergency Department complaining of a nose bleed for the past 3 hours. He could not recall any history of trauma. The patient's history was significant for recently diagnosed phlebitis in his left lower leg for which he had been taking warfarin for the past 6 weeks. He stated that his most recent prothrombin time was "just fine." He also had hypertension, controlled with metoprolol. There was no history of prior nosebleeds, and the patient denied headache, chest pain, shortness of breath, dizziness, bruising, or any change in bowel or bladder.

Examination revealed a man sitting holding a bloody handkerchief over his nose with some gagging. Supine vital signs were blood pressure of 110/80, pulse 80/minute and regular, respirations 18/minute, and oral temperature 98.0° F. Excluding the nose, general physical examination was unremarkable. No ecchymoses were noted.

A blood clot was noted in the left nostril, with no active bleeding from either nares. There was a small amount of dried blood along the right septum. Inspection of the oropharynx with a tongue blade revealed a large clot hanging down from the nasopharynx.

Laboratory studies revealed a hematocrit of 42%, platelet count of 230,000, and a prothrombin time of 17 seconds.

DIAGNOSTIC CLUES:

1. The patient's standing blood pressure was 96/70 with a pulse of 80/minute.

2. The clot was removed from the left nasal cavity, revealing a small arterial bleeding blood vessel from the anterior septum.

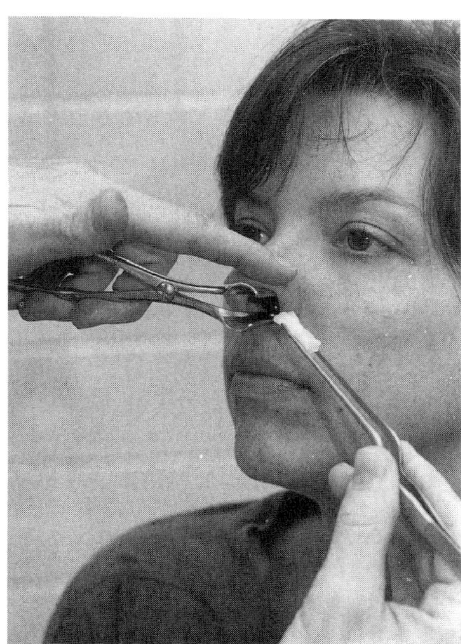

QUESTIONS:

1. What is the diagnosis?

2. In comparing anterior versus posterior epistaxis, which is more common and which produces significant blood loss?

3. What should be done when a patient presents to the Emergency Department with a history of epistaxis that has stopped by the time of the physician's evaluation?

4. Should this patient's prothrombin time prolongation have been reversed to control epistaxis? What if his prothrombin time were 27 seconds?

5. Describe the management of epistaxis, including the use of vasoconstrictors, cautery, and anterior and posterior packing.

ANSWERS:

1. The diagnosis in this case is spontaneous (nontraumatic) anterior epistaxis. Although there are many reasons a nose may bleed, in most cases a specific etiology cannot be identified.

2. The blood supply to the nose involves extensive anastomosis of blood vessels, with the sphenopalatine and anterior ethmoidal arteries being the most important. However, from the standpoint of the emergency physician, there are two types of nasal bleeding: anterior and posterior. It is important to identify the site of the bleed since the location will dictate treatment.

Anterior bleeds account for the large majority of nosebleeds (close to 90%), usually originating at the anterior aspect of the nasal septum in a region known as Kiesselbach's area.

Posterior bleeds are usually difficult, if not impossible, to visualize and often are not suspected until anterior packing fails to control nasal hemorrhage. Posterior epistaxis is usually seen in elderly patients with a history of hypertension and/or atherosclerotic vascular disease.

While posterior epistaxis is more commonly associated with significant hemorrhage, an anterior nosebleed can also result in hemodynamic instability.

3. When a patient comes to the Emergency Department with a history of a nosebleed that is controlled, it is still important to obtain a careful history and physical examination including vital signs. Bleeding will often recur. In a patient with a compromised cardiovascular status, this could precipitate a syncopal event and has even been reported to be the terminal event in elderly patients with coronary insufficiency.

A history should be obtained in regard to duration, frequency, and amount of bleeding; history of trauma; and use of alcohol or drugs. After the general physical examination is completed, the patient and physician should be gowned to prepare for examination of the nose. The equipment required should be readily available: head lamp or mirror, nasal speculum, suction with a Fraser tip, bayonet forceps, cotton or gauze pledgets, cautery, and topical vasoconstrictors/anesthetics. The patient should sit upright and blow his nose to help remove clots.

The physician should look first in the nares where the patient initially noted bleeding, opening the nasal speculum vertically, without compressing the septum (see illustration). The physician should proceed in a systematic manner, starting at the anterior inferior quadrant of the nasal septum, where most anterior bleeds occur. If no active bleeding is

seen after clot removal, areas which appear friable can
tip applicator. This maneuver will not elicit bleeding in n
still no bleeding evident, the patient should be observe
aware that cyclic bleeding is characteristic of posterior

4. In almost all cases, anterior epistaxis can be con
regardless of the prolongation of the prothrombin time.
generally utilized for relatively significant indications, th
warfarin dose to achieve the desired therapeutic level. T
epistaxis of life-threatening proportions that require reve
fresh frozen plasma (note that vitamin K will not immed

5. In general, the bleeding point should be controlled with the least possible manipulation and discomfort to the patient. After ensuring the patency of the airway and hemodynamic stability, one can proceed with local treatment of the nosebleed. If there is any question of hemodynamic instability, an intravenous catheter should be placed and crystalloids infused.

If an anterior bleeding point can be readily identified on the initial examination, the area should be anesthetized with a topical anesthetic and then cauterized. Usually a silver nitrate stick applied carefully to the bleeding site for approximately 20 seconds will suffice. It is important to remove clots, because these will inhibit coagulation of the region to be cauterized. Electrocautery has also been utilized, but this has a higher incidence of septal perforation.

Occasionally, bleeding may be too brisk to allow cauterization. The judicious use of a cotton pledget soaked with a topical vasoconstrictor such as 4% cocaine, epinephrine (1:1000), or phenylephrine 0.5%, applied over the bleeding site for 5 to 10 minutes will usually slow the bleeding enough to allow cauterization of the bleeding site. If these measures control the bleeding, the patient should be observed for another 30 minutes. Careful discharge instructions should be given to the patient, instructing him not to blow his nose for the next 48 hours, to sneeze with his mouth open, not to use aspirin or nonsteroidal antiinflammatory drugs for one week, and to use saline nose drops or a weak vasoconstrictor for 1 week. The patient should also be advised that bleeding may recur (10 to 20% incidence).

If cautery is unsuccessful, one can attempt to control the bleeding by injecting approximately 1 cc of 1% lidocaine with epinephrine (1:100,000) directly beneath the bleeding site.

rs do not control bleeding, the next step is anterior packing. If done usually control most anterior bleeds. However, it is not without

packing will occlude drainage from the nasal sinuses as well as cause the significant discomfort. Anterior packing requires 4 to 6 feet of 1/4- to 1/2-inch e impregnated with bacitracin or neosporin ointment carefully layered with bayonet rceps. Remember, the purpose of packing is to apply pressure to every "nook and cranny," so the nares must be packed solid. An additional consideration is that since the anterior portion of the septum is cartilage and displaces easily, both nares may have to be packed.

If packing controls bleeding, the pack will need to stay in place for 3 to 5 days. The patient should be placed on an antibiotic, i.e., amoxicillin, cephalosporin, or erythromycin as well as a decongestant and analgesic. Arrangements should be made for the patient to be seen in 24 hours. Before the patient is discharged, the posterior pharynx must be inspected for bleeding. If one is uncertain of continued bleeding, the patient should gargle followed by inspection of the pharynx.

Otolaryngologic consultation is warranted in all patients requiring posterior packing. Treatment of posterior epistaxis will require compression of the posterior nasopharynx, which can be accomplished with various modalities including a posterior pack, a Foley catheter (16 to 18 French), or a commercially available balloon device. Not only must these patients be hospitalized but for the first 24 hours they need to be in an intensive care setting, since they are prone to hypoxia and arrhythmias. Additional intervention, such as surgical ligation of the artery and embolization, may be required in refractory or recurrent bleeding.

One final point is that packing should be avoided if possible in patients with known blood dyscrasias. Oxycell or Gelfoam often proves useful in this setting.

PEARLS:

1. When an anterior bleed is brisk or forms a clot occluding one of the nares, blood can travel around the posterior portion of the nasal septum, creating the appearance of bleeding from both nostrils. Always inquire from which side the bleeding initially appeared. This will usually be the site of the bleed.

2. Check the posterior pharynx for clots, as these can be irritating to the patient and precipitate gagging.

3. If there is a history of trauma, carefully search for a septal hematoma. This results from extravasation of blood between the cartilage and perichondrium and will appear as a

bulge in the septum. Septal hematomas must be promptly incised to avoid destruction and infection of the septum.

4. Salt pork (cured pork side meat) possesses hemostatic properties and is often useful in patients with blood dyscrasias, particularly leukemic patients and patients with low platelet counts. Gelfoam and Oxycell are also useful in this setting.

5. Unilateral nasal bleeding in a patient who also complains of nasal obstruction may indicate a neoplasm within the nose, nasopharynx, or nasal sinuses.

6. In patients with "occult" nasal bleeding where no source can be found, make sure the bleeding isn't from the respiratory or gastrointestinal tracts. The converse also applies--consider nasal bleeding in hematemesis and melena.

PITFALLS:

1. Never fail to obtain postural vital signs in a patient who relates significant bleeding. However, be aware that many medications, especially antihypertensives and psychiatric medications can produce postural hypotension, while beta blockers can blunt the expected tachycardic response.

2. There is no need to routinely order a hematocrit, platelet count, and bleeding parameters in every case of epistaxis. Epistaxis is rarely the sole initial manifestation of a bleeding diathesis. Allow the history and physical examination to dictate the need for these tests.

3. Don't forget to use the proper dosages of topical vasoconstrictors and anesthetics. These medications are well absorbed from the nasal mucosa and can precipitate cardiac ischemia, arrhythmias, and seizures if not used properly.

4. When inserting gauze for an anterior pack, do not insert the lead end into the nose first, as it can fall down into the pharynx and possibly cause airway obstruction and discomfort.

5. Do not precipitously lower a patient's blood pressure. Hypertension is rarely a cause of epistaxis. Often the patient's blood pressure will be elevated secondary to anxiety over the nosebleed.

6. Do not fail to examine the posterior pharynx after "control" of an anterior bleed.

REFERENCES:

Charles R, Corrigan E. Epistaxis and hypertension. Postgrad Med 1977;53:260-261.

Heywood BB, Davis RB, Yonkers AJ. Treatment of epistaxis with porcine stripped packing. Trans Am Acad Ophthamol Otolaryngol 1977;82:255-257.

Kirckner JA. Epistaxis. N Engl J Med 1982;307(18):1126-1128.

Maceri DR. Nasal trauma. In: Cummings CW, Krause CJ, eds. Otolaryngology--head and neck surgery. St. Louis: CV Mosby, 1986:614-623.

Rosnagle RS. Epistaxis. In: English GM, ed. Otolaryngology. Philadelphia: JB Lippincott, 1990;chapter 25.

Votey S, Dudley JP. Emergency nose and throat procedures. Emerg Med Clin North Am 1989;7(1):131-140.

EYE TRAUMA

Case 23:

INITIAL VISIT:

A 30-year-old father presented to the Emergency Department 2 hours after his young son inadvertently scratched his eye. He developed immediate eye pain that seemed worse with blinking. He stated that he thought his vision was decreased in the right eye, although he did not bring his glasses. His past medical history was unremarkable. He was not taking any medication and could not recall his last tetanus shot.

The nurse could not perform a visual acuity examination on the injured right eye, because the patient stated that he had too much pain, tearing, and blurriness. Inspection and palpation revealed mild injection of the cornea, and normal bone and surrounding soft tissue structures. There was increased tearing from the affected right eye, but no purulent discharge was noted. The lids were everted, and no foreign bodies were seen. Penlight exam revealed a flat and clear anterior chamber, and the pupil reaction was normal for both direct and consensual reflexes.

After the instillation of a topical anesthetic, visual acuity was determined with the aid of a pinhole card and found to be 20/20 in the unaffected left eye and 20/30 in the injured right eye. Old records revealed that the patient had received a tetanus booster 5 years ago.

The physician applied fluorescein to the eye with a moistened fluorescein strip and applied a Wood's lamp to illuminate the eye.

DIAGNOSTIC CLUE:

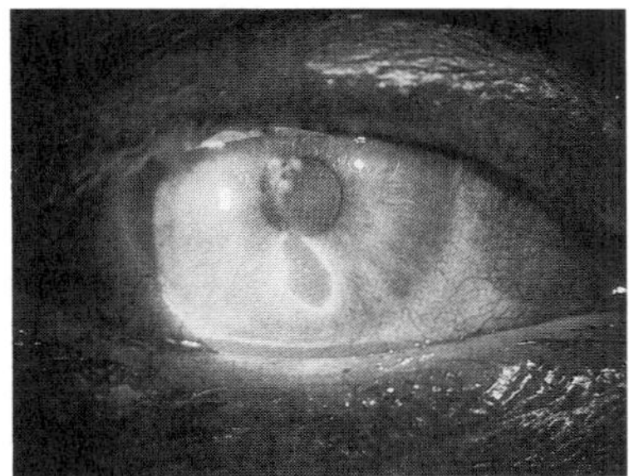

QUESTIONS:

1. Discuss the initial approach to the patient with an injured eye in the Emergency Department.

2. What is the diagnosis in this patient?

3. What treatment is indicated?

4. What are the potential complications of this injury?

5. What should be the initial disposition of this patient?

RETURN VISIT:

The patient returned to the Emergency Department 2 months later stating that "I must have scratched my eye again." On further questioning, he stated that while hammering a nail into the wall, he struck a glancing blow to the nail and "a piece of something flew into my eye." He experienced pain similar to when he scratched his eye 2 months earlier. This time the patient brought his glasses and his corrected vision was 20/30 in the unaffected right eye and 20/60 in the painful left eye. On close inspection, the right pupil was noted to have an irregular contour, having a "pear-shape" appearance and not reacting to light. On slit lamp examination, it appeared that a small amount of the iris was prolapsing from a scleral laceration at 8 o'clock.

DIAGNOSTIC CLUES:

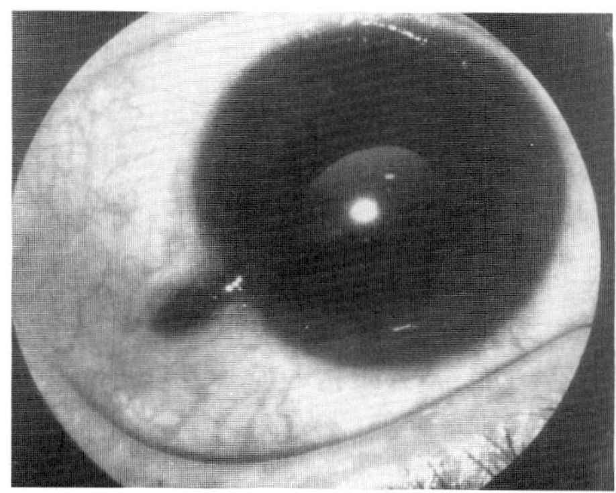

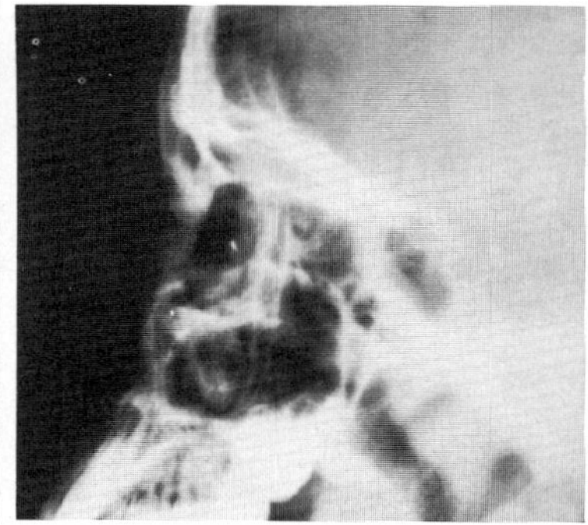

QUESTIONS:

6. What is the diagnosis?

7. How does one make this diagnosis? How important is the visual acuity exam in making this diagnosis?

8. What management is indicated in the Emergency Department and how urgent is ophthalmologic consultation?

ANSWERS:

1. When a patient comes to the Emergency Department with an eye complaint, it is the responsibility of the initial care provider to differentiate between a potentially serious vision-threatening problem and a less serious situation. It is often this initial care that will determine the ultimate outcome when dealing with eye injuries. As in most medical problems, the history will help to predict the type of damage to expect. The history should include a detailed description of how the eye injury occurred, subsequent symptoms, what first aid and treatment has already been rendered, previous history of eye disease (including eyeglass or contact lens wear), general medical history, current medications and allergies, and current tetanus status.

Visual acuity should always be part of the initial examination. If the patient has his glasses, test corrected vision. If the patient does not have his glasses, an approximation of corrected vision can be made by having him look through a pinhole punched in a piece of paper. Even in major eye injuries the ability to detect light and to tell its direction when tested from each quadrant is important. The only exception to testing visual acuity first is with chemical burns to the eye.

The remainder of the examination will be dictated by the history and visual acuity, but basically, as in this case, one should check pupillary responses, extraocular movements, and lids and lashes and then proceed to the slit lamp examination and funduscopic exam. If there is obvious rupture of the optic globe, no further manipulation of the eye should be done.

2. The diagnosis here is corneal abrasion. Typically, this injury is caused by a fingernail or similar object (e.g., tree branch, paper, contact lens) scratching the eye. The patient will usually complain of a foreign body sensation as well as photophobia and tearing.

3. After instillation of anesthetic drops, such as proparacaine or tetracaine, stain the eye with fluorescein. Epithelial loss (corneal abrasion) can be confirmed with a Wood's lamp, but it is best to examine the eye with a slit lamp in order to adequately view the anterior chamber. Although individual patients vary greatly, spasm of the ciliary muscle often occurs after corneal abrasion, producing significant pain, and a short-acting cycloplegic agent such as cyclopentolate will often provide relief. In addition, since this "open wound" is somewhat susceptible to infection, prophylactic topical antibiotic ointments or drops can be instilled (there is some controversy as to whether ointments retard healing).

Patching, if done properly, is believed to be helpful, relieving the pain caused by continual blinking and preventing impairment of reepithelialization. While patching seems like a simple task, if done improperly it can aggravate the problem. When patching, have the patient tightly close the eye, fold the first eye patch in two, and apply a second patch over this for a three-layer effect. The tape strips are then stretched diagonally from the center of the forehead to the cheek bone (the skin can be carefully prepped with benzoin beforehand).

What if a foreign body is still present? If the foreign body appears superficial, i.e., not embedded, one can attempt to irrigate it off the cornea. If it is not deeply embedded, i.e., not deeper than Bowman's capsule, and the emergency physician has been properly trained, removal with a commercial spud or a fine-gauge needle (25- to 30-gauge) using a small syringe or cotton-tipped applicator as a handle can be attempted. However, it cannot be overemphasized that the emergency caregiver must always be wary of the potential for an intraocular or intraorbital foreign body, and if there is any question, an ophthalmologist needs to be consulted. Contrary to what one may expect, it is very difficult to penetrate the sclera or cornea. Also keep in mind that the removal of a foreign body is not the end of treatment, as a rust ring often develops even after removal of a metal foreign body.

4. Corneal abrasions should heal without problems in 24 to 72 hours. However, as with any wound, complications can occur, such as secondary bacterial infections which may lead to a bacterial ulcer or hypopyon. These usually present as increasing pain and purulent discharge. Slightly later, usually 3 to 6 days after the injury, the patient can develop posttraumatic iritis and present with pain, decreased vision, meiosis, and perilimbal injection. One final complication is recurrent corneal abrasions, which are believed to result from imperfect healing of the epithelium.

5. Follow-up is just as important as the history, physical exam, and treatment. All patients with an increase in pain or a decrease in vision should be instructed to seek immediate medical care, regardless of the initial ocular complaint. Regular follow-up for eye trauma should be arranged with an ophthalmologist or the patient's family physician in 24 to 48 hours. Any patient who is patched should be instructed not to drive or operate heavy machinery.

6. When communicating the type of injury to the ophthalmologist, it is important to use the proper terminology, so that he or she can establish a proper mental picture of the injury. Laceration implies a defect in the cornea or sclera caused by a sharp instrument, such as a knife or high-velocity missile (such as a metal fragment projected from a hammer or chisel). Injury from blunt trauma of sufficient force to cause a disruption of the sclera or cornea is referred to as a rupture. If either of these injuries traverses the full thickness of the sclera or cornea and enters the intraocular cavity, then this is diagnosed as a perforation. This patient has a corneal laceration with most likely a global perforation.

7. Suspecting the injury is possibly the most challenging aspect of perforation injuries of the eye. It is imperative that a detailed description of how the eye injury occurred be obtained. The history of something hitting a patient's eye after using a hammer or chisel suggests an intraocular foreign body until proven otherwise. The classic appearance of the eye in this situation is a shallow anterior chamber and a teardrop-shaped pupil that points toward the perforation. One should be aware that with many of these injuries there may not be eye pain.

Although diminished visual acuity is an important finding, if the foreign body is not interfering with the visual axis, visual acuity may be undisturbed. Furthermore, there may be minimal evidence of external damage to the eye; a small metal fragment may penetrate the eye, causing internal damage but seal the entry wound with no prolapse. Often, intraocular foreign bodies will not even be present on direct ophthalmoscopy. Determination of the need for x-rays, sonograms, or computed tomography should be done in conjunction with the consulting ophthalmologist.

8. The primary task of the emergency physician is to suspect the diagnosis and protect the eye from further harm while obtaining ophthalmologic consultation. A metal shield should be placed over the affected eye. If a metal shield is not available, a substitute can be fashioned with a plastic foam cup. No further examination or manipulation should be done once the diagnosis is suspected. This includes no ointments or other medication placed in the eye. The measurement of intraocular pressures is contraindicated.

The patient should be kept NPO in anticipation of surgery, and analgesics and antiemetics should be liberally prescribed to prevent restlessness, nausea, and vomiting, which may cause further harm. Tetanus status should be updated as necessary. The consulting ophthalmologist should determine initial antibiotic coverage. Studies support the concept that early surgery provides better results. If an ophthalmologist cannot be available within several hours and the patient is neurologically stable, consideration should be given to transferring the patient to the nearest eye trauma center by the fastest means possible.

PEARLS:

1. When a patient has forgotten his or her glasses, visual acuity can be checked with a pinhole card.

2. A simple diagnostic test for superficial eye injuries (i.e., superficial abrasion, conjunctivitis) is that pain is almost completely relieved by topical anesthetics, whereas the pain of iritis or deeper structures will not be relieved.

3. Swelling in and around the periorbital structures can mask signs of a blow-out fracture. Any patient with significant periorbital blunt trauma should have plain roentgenograms.

4. A pattern of vertical scratch marks on the cornea indicates a foreign body entrapped on the conjunctival surface of the upper lid.

5. A fourth of all hyphemas are associated with another ocular injury. These should always be referred to an ophthalmologist for urgent consultation.

6. The history of something hitting a patient's eye while hammering or chiseling suggests an intraocular foreign body until proven otherwise.

PITFALLS:

1. Never prescribe or dispense topical anesthetics to the patient. These retard healing and the patient can inadvertently injure himself.

2. Use fluorescein strips, not solution. Studies have demonstrated that fluorescein solution is a good medium for growth of Pseudomonas species.

3. Except for chemical burns, always check visual acuity first. Dilating the pupil or instilling drops into the eye may adversely affect vision.

4. Never assume a red eye is just conjunctivitis. Particularly in children, foreign bodies can be hidden under the lid, presenting as a red eye.

5. Do not allow a patient who has had one eye patched to drive or operate machinery. Depth perception is lost and injury may result.

6. Do not use Neosporin solutions in the eye. These cause a sensitizing reaction in up to 15% of patients.

REFERENCES:

Born CP. Ocular injuries--treat or refer. Postgrad Med 1983;73:311-317.

Eagling EA. Perforating injuries of the eye. Br J Ophthalmol 1976;60:732-736.

Elkington AR, Khaw PT. injuries to the eye. Brit Med J 1988;297:122-125.

Hoffman JR, Nehaus RW, Baylis HI. Penetrating orbital trauma. Am J Emerg Med 1983;1:22-27.

Manners R. Ocular trauma. Practitioner 1990; 234:96-100.

Matthews J, Zun LS. Ophthalmologic emergencies and ocular trauma. Emerg Clin North Am 1988; 6(1).

A YOUNG MAN WITH A BULLET TO THE CHEST

Case 24:

A young male was bought to the Emergency Department after sustaining a single gunshot wound to the left side of the chest. The paramedics reported that the patient was pale and diaphoretic at the scene with initial vital signs of systolic blood pressure 80, heart rate 140/minute, and labored respirations at a rate of 32/minute, and decreased breath sounds over the left side of the chest. Police told the medics that the patient was shot approximately 10 minutes before their arrival; transport time to the hospital was approximately 5 minutes. Supplemental oxygen was provided by a high-flow face mask, and two 14-gauge intravenous catheters were started in the left and right antecubital fossae en route.

On arrival in the Emergency Department, the patient was verbally unresponsive, respirations were shallow, with decreased breath sounds over the left hemithorax. A carotid pulse was barely palpable. On quick inspection, the neck veins were noted to be nondistended, and a single entrance wound was noted on the left side of the chest at the fifth intercostal space, midclavicular line. No exit wound was noted. No other injuries were apparent.

DIAGNOSTIC CLUE:

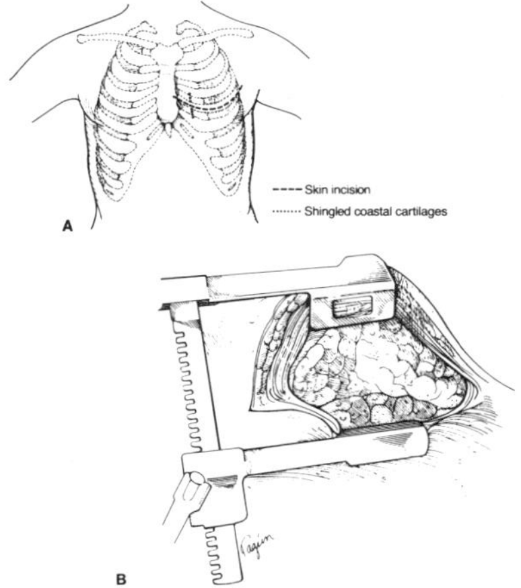

QUESTIONS:

1. Discuss the prehospital care of penetrating wounds to the chest.

2. What injuries are immediately life-threatening in a patient with penetrating chest trauma?

3. What should be the initial steps in the management of this patient?

4. What role does emergency thoracotomy play in treatment of penetrating chest trauma?

ANSWERS:

1. Prehospital care has come a long way from the days when hearses doubled as ambulances. With the advent of standards of training for emergency medical technicians and paramedics, designation of trauma centers, and a more rapid response time, patients who would have been dead at the scene now survive to hospital discharge. Three factors are largely responsible for determining outcome: (1) the type of injury or constellation of injuries, (2) a patient's physiologic reserve (the older the patient and the more serious the preexisting disease, the less the reserve), and (3) time lapse between injury and definitive medical intervention. Since it is difficult to influence the first two factors, it is often the third factor that determines survival of traumatic insult.

Especially with penetrating trauma, delivery of the patient in a maximally expedient manner to an experienced trauma team is of utmost importance. In penetrating chest trauma, standard interventions such as MAST (military antishock trousers) and external cardiac massage have been found to be ineffective. Only the "basics," including maintenance of the airway, stabilizing the neck, and control of hemorrhage should be performed at the scene. The patient should otherwise be transported in the most rapid manner. With the exception of cases of patient entrapment at the scene, prehospital intravenous lines should be initiated during transport.

2. The majority of patients with penetrating chest trauma will not require formal surgical intervention. Prompt and immediate correction of several life-threatening injuries can prevent irreversible shock leading to death. Penetrating injuries to the thorax generally cause shock by one of three mechanisms: ventilatory impairment, hypovolemia, and/or cardiac (pump) failure.

While respiratory compromise is usually obvious on physical exam, it may be more difficult to distinguish hypovolemia from pump failure. The classic distinguishing feature between these two causes of shock is central venous pressure, usually reflected in the neck veins. If the neck veins are flat, then hypovolemia may be a contributing factor. However, if the neck veins are distended initially or if they become full during volume restoration before hypotension has fully resolved, then there may be a cardiac component to the patient's condition.

There are five life-threatening conditions that may be associated with penetrating chest trauma: (1) open pneumothorax, (2) tension pneumothorax, (3) massive hemothorax, (4) cardiac wound/cardiac tamponade, and (5) air embolism.

While most penetrating injuries to the thorax will seal themselves, larger defects will remain open producing an open pneumothorax. It is generally believed if the opening in the chest wall is two-thirds or greater than the diameter of the trachea, air flow will follow the path of least resistance and enter through the chest wall defect. This will lead to rapid equilibration between atmospheric and pleural pressures, causing ventilatory impairment. Immediate management includes closing the defect with an occlusive dressing taped on three edges (if all four edges are taped, an open pneumothorax can be converted into a closed tension pneumothorax). Once the patient is in the Emergency Department, a tube thoracostomy is performed on the affected hemithorax remote from the wound. A more definitive surgical procedure to close the defect may be required.

A tension pneumothorax is created when air is allowed to enter the pleural cavity but cannot escape. This eventually leads to a high pleural pressure and collapse of the lung with some respiratory compromise. However, the main reason patients with tension pneumothorax die is circulatory compromise. When pressure develops in the involved hemithorax, the heart is pushed to the opposite side. Since the superior and inferior vena cava are relatively fixed structures, if the heart is displaced far enough, the venous return (preload) from the superior and inferior vena cava is impaired, reducing cardiac output and producing shock.

The clinical signs of tension pneumothorax are respiratory distress with decreased breath sounds and hyperresonance to percussion on the affected side. There may be neck vein distention and deviation of the trachea away from the affected side. Temporizing treatment involves needle decompression with a 16-gauge needle into the second intercostal space at the midclavicular line of the affected hemithorax. Definitive treatment involves placement of a chest tube into the fifth intercostal space, anterior to the midaxillary line in the involved side of the chest (see illustration).

The term massive hemothorax implies greater than 1500 cc of blood loss into the involved chest cavity. The patient presents in shock with decreased or absent breath sounds on the affected side and dullness to percussion of the involved hemithorax. Neck veins may or may not be distended. While loss of ipsilateral lung function compromises respiration, the main problem here is exsanguination. Therefore, treatment should be directed toward volume replacement with crystalloids and type-specific blood. Once volume is partially restored, a tube thoracostomy can be performed on the affected side. An autotransfusion device, which utilizes blood from the chest cavity, can be most useful in this setting.

Any patient in shock with a penetrating wound of the chest between the midclavicular line on the right and the midaxillary line on the left should be presumed to have a cardiac wound until proven otherwise. Penetrating cardiac injuries usually present in one of three ways: (1) a small wound which seals spontaneously, (2) penetration of the heart and pericardium with rapid exsanguination into the thorax, and (3) penetration with a relatively intact pericardium resulting in tamponade. Often the type of injury is influenced by the instrument of violence, viz., stab wounds tend to cause limited injury while gunshot wounds of the pericardium and cardiac chambers are often quite large with hemorrhage dominating the clinical presentation.

Since the pericardial sac is relatively inelastic, as little as 60 cc of blood and clots in the pericardium can present as cardiac tamponade. Beck's classic triad of distended neck veins, muffled heart tones, and decreased pulse pressure is associated with cardiac tamponade. In reality, these classic findings are often absent. Neck veins may be flat from hypovolemia, and heart sounds are often difficult to evaluate in a noisy Emergency Department. The key to diagnosis is a high index of suspicion.

In cardiac tamponade secondary to trauma, blood entrapped in the pericardium creates positive pressure around the heart, compressing the cardiac chambers and preventing filling of the heart. Early in tamponade, treatment is directed toward rapid volume infusion in an attempt to overcome the increased right ventricular pressures caused by the tamponade. However, volume infusion is only temporizing. In the past, pericardio-centesis was the next step in management of a patient with suspected pericardial tamponade who was hypotensive and unresponsive to fluid administration. Many trauma surgeons now perform subxyphoid pericardiotomy or thoracotomy because of the high false-negative and false-positive rates of pericardiocentesis. Any patient with a positive pericardiocentesis or exploration will require a thoracotomy for definitive management.

Recently, air embolism has been recognized as a complication of thoracic trauma, particularly with penetrating injuries. The embolism results from a traumatic fistula formed between a bronchus and a pulmonary vein. Normally, the pressure gradient directs flow from the pulmonary vein to the bronchus, but if the patient is intubated and placed on positive pressure ventilation, this gradient is reversed, forcing air from the bronchus to the pulmonary vein. From the pulmonary vein, the embolism makes its way to the left ventricle and can then be injected into the systemic circulation, where it can lodge in the coronary or cerebral arterial beds. While this is a very difficult diagnosis to make, it should be suspected in a patient who has cardiovascular collapse after endotracheal intubation or in a patient with chest trauma without obvious head trauma who acutely develops focal or lateralizing neurologic signs. Treatment involves emergency thoracotomy with cross-clamping of the involved hilum, aspiration of the left atrium, left ventricle, and ascending aorta for two to three heartbeats to try to increase the afterload and attempt to push the air embolus through the coronary vessels.

3. As previously stated, the emergency care of any patient always begins with the ABC's of airway, breathing, and circulation. This care needs to be preconceived and prioritized, particularly with trauma patients. While the primary survey is being conducted, resuscitative procedures are performed simultaneously to minimize morbidity and mortality.

Since this patient is in profound shock, intubation is the preferred route for control of the airway. Once the airway is secured, the mechanics of breathing need to be addressed. In this scenario there is a good chance of a pneumothorax and/or hemothorax. Early evacuation of the pleural space by a tube thoracostomy on the left side may improve the respiratory and hemodynamic status of the patient. An autotransfuser, which recycles blood from the chest should be connected to the chest tube. Remember that the greatest blood loss is usually during the initial insertion of the tube into the chest.

Intravenous access has already been obtained in this patient. A general guideline is that for wounds below the nipples, upper body access is usually indicated, while with wounds above the nipples, lower extremity access also should be obtained.

A patient presenting in extremis, such as this patient, has generally lost at least 40% of his blood volume. Isotonic electrolyte solutions are used initially to provide transient intravascular expansion. Ideally, the best fluid of replacement is whole blood, but because of its limited supply, packed red blood cells are usually given. No arbitrary rule for the amount of blood required can be applied, because of the variable amount of initial and ongoing hemorrhage as well as changes in venous capacitance. A central venous line may prove valuable in judging fluid therapy by allowing the physician to monitor central venous pressures.

Subsequent management will be determined by the hemodynamic stability of the patient and capabilities of the Emergency Department and staff. Hypotensive patients with penetrating chest trauma who fail to respond to volume infusion usually do so because of inability to keep up with the ongoing hemorrhage or presence of a tamponade or tension pneumothorax. In any patient with penetrating chest trauma who is in shock with distended neck veins or a tension penumothorax, initial management is directed toward a tension pneumothorax, i.e., immediate decompression of the affected hemithorax, with a chest tube. If the patient's condition continues to deteriorate and the neck veins are either initially distended or become distended despite a properly performed tube thoracostomy, the next consideration should be cardiac tamponade.

If cardiac tamponade is suspected and the patient is hemodynamically unstable despite intubation, tube thoracostomy, and fluid resuscitation sufficient to raise central venous pressure above 20 cm H_2O, it is best whenever possible to transport the patient to an operating room where a subxyphoid pericardial window can be performed. If the patient deteriorates to the point of cardiac arrest, then an immediate thoracotomy is indicated.

4. Despite the fact that Emergency Department thoracotomy is considered a radical procedure in the management of a patient with chest trauma, thoracotomy is being employed with increasing frequency in trauma centers. While there is still much controversy related to this procedure, its indications are becoming more clearly defined. In a select group of patients (principally but not exclusively patients with penetrating chest trauma) an emergency thoracotomy can be lifesaving.

The decision to initiate an Emergency Department thoracotomy is multifactorial. It should be based on the mechanism of injury, anatomic location of the wound, time span from the moment of injury to presentation, and personnel available. In general, the best candidates are those victims of penetrating chest trauma who present with some signs of life, while the worst prognosis is for victims of blunt trauma without vital signs.

The principal objectives of a thoracotomy are to: (1) release a pericardial tamponade, (2) control massive intrathoracic hemorrhage, (3) provide access for open cardiac massage, and (4) permit temporary occlusion of the descending thoracic aorta to help redistribute blood flow to the heart and brain. It is generally agreed that if at all possible the patient should be stabilized and transported to the operating room where more optimal conditions exist.

Immediate thoracotomy in the Emergency Department is indicated for the patient with penetrating chest trauma with no vital signs in the Emergency Department but recent vital signs in the past 5 minutes (i.e., palpable pulse or respirations) or the patient who is rapidly deteriorating in the Emergency Department. It is difficult to analyze the success rate of emergency thoracotomy because of the various criteria used to classify patients based on their initial presentation as well as differences for stab wounds versus gunshot wounds, single chamber versus multiple chamber involvement, and differences in organ system involvement.

If an emergency thoracotomy is performed, there must be a qualified surgeon available for definitive repair. Thoracotomy should not be performed in patients without vital signs at the scene of the accident, victims of blunt trauma without vital signs in the Emergency Department, and patients who are not otherwise salvageable (e.g., a patient with a gunshot wound of the head and chest in whom the head wound is fatal).

Before a thoracotomy is performed, central oxygenation must be restored, preferably by endotracheal intubation, and fluid resuscitation begun. Resuscitative efforts will be fruitless unless one is able to reverse hypoxia and hypovolemia. It may also be beneficial to place the patient in Trendelenberg's position to decrease the risk of a systemic air embolus.

Traditionally, a left anterolateral incision through the fifth intercostal space from the sternum to the posteroaxillary line has been utilized. In the female, the incision is centered over the inframammary fold. The left sided thoracotomy provides access to not only the heart but also the aorta. After the incision is made, a rib retractor is placed in the chest and the pericardium is opened in the craniocaudal direction medial and parallel to the phrenic nerve. With injuries involving both hemithoraces, a median sternotomy is the best approach to opening the chest.

Initial attempts at controlling bleeding from the heart should be with digital pressure. Only a physician experienced in cardiac repair should attempt to suture the heart wound. In some instances a Foley catheter can be passed into the ventricle, inflating the balloon with sterile saline and applying gentle traction to stop the bleeding. Bleeding from the atria cannot usually be controlled with digital pressure and will usually require an atraumatic vascular clamp. Other procedures may include cross-clamping of the aorta, clamping of the pulmonary hilum, and open cardiac massage. As soon as possible, the patient should be taken to the operating room for definitive surgical repair.

PEARLS:

1. Less than 15% of chest injuries require early surgical intervention--the majority can be controlled with bedside procedures.

2. While both a pneumothorax and hemothorax present with decreased or absent breath sounds on the affected side, a pneumothorax usually demonstrates hyperresonance to percussion, while a hemothorax usually presents as dullness to percussion.

3. In patients with penetrating wounds of the heart. The most commonly wounded chamber is the right ventricle by virtue of its anterior position; this is followed by the left ventricle, right atrium, and finally the left atrium.

4. If a patient arrests immediately after endotracheal intubation is performed, suspect one of the following: (1) inadequate preoxygenation, (2) endotracheal tube not in the trachea, (3) tension pneumothorax, or (4) systemic air embolus.

PITFALLS:

1. Tension pneumothorax is a clinical, not radiologic diagnosis. Whenever a tension pneumothorax is suspected, immediate decompression of the affected chest cavity is indicated.

2. Contrary to traditional teaching, pericardial blood can clot in the pericardial sac and interfere with aspiration. Therefore, a negative pericardiocentesis does not rule out a tamponade. Moreover, with fresh bleeding into the pericardium the blood aspirated will not be defibrinated and will clot, yielding a false result.

3. In acute cardiac tamponade secondary to trauma, the classic Beck's triad of distended neck veins, muffled heart tones, and hypotension will be present less than 40% of the time.

4. Any penetrating wound at or below the level of the nipples may pierce the diaphragm and enter the abdominal cavity.

5. If performing open cardiac massage, use the palms and volar aspects of the hand and not the fingertips. Cardiac muscle is fragile and can be easily damaged.

REFERENCES:

Cogbill TH, Moore EE, Millkan JS, Cleveland HC. Rationale for selective application of emergency thoracotomy in trauma. J Trauma 1983;23(6):453-460.

Feliciano DV, Mattox KL. Indications, techniques, and pitfalls of emergency center thoracotomy. Surg Rounds 1981;(Dec.):32-40.

Jacobs LM, Sinclair A, Beiser A, et al. Prehospital advanced life support: benefits in trauma. J Trauma 1984;24:8-13.

Mattox KL, Bickell W, Pepe PE, et al. Prospective MAST study in 911 patients. J Trauma 1989;29:1104-1112.

Roberge RJ, Ivatory RR, Stahl W, et al. Emergency Department thoracotomy for penetrating trauma: predictive value of patient classification. Am J Emerg Med 1986;42(2):129-135.

Yee ES, Vernier ED, Thomas AN. Management of air embolism in blunt and penetrating thoracic trauma. J Thorac Surg 1983;85:661-668.

AN ASTHMATIC WITH DIARRHEA

Case 25:

A 63-year-old white male with a long-standing history of asthma presented to the Emergency Department complaining of 8 days of abdominal pain, anorexia, nausea, vomiting, and watery diarrhea. He described up to six watery, brown bowel movements/day and denied any red blood in the stool or melena. He had vomited several times in the past 2 days and stated the vomitus contained partially digested food without red blood or "coffee grounds." He described the abdominal pain as diffuse and crampy in quality. He denied fever and stated no other member of his family had similar complaints. He had no recent travel history.

The patient's past medical history was remarkable for asthma since childhood. He had never been intubated, but had frequent severe bouts of asthma throughout his life and had been steroid-dependent for the past 5 years. He additionally stated he had been diagnosed with pulmonary tuberculosis 20 years earlier and received treatment for one year. In addition, he had been diagnosed with hypertension and non-insulin dependent diabetes mellitus 10 years earlier.

His medications included Theodur 300 mg bid, prednisone 10 mg daily, Proventil inhaler qid, Vanceril inhaler qid, Alupent nebulizer bid, nifedipine 20 tid, hydrochlorothiazide 50 mg daily, and glyburide 2.5 mg bid. He denied any recent increase in usage of bronchodilators, stating that his asthma had been so well-controlled of late that he had been able to sharply decrease his medication usage. He denied any history of cigarette smoking and stated he drank alcohol on rare occasions.

On physical examination, he was an obese white male with pale skin who appeared diaphoretic and ill at ease. His blood pressure was 100/60, pulse 120/minute and regular, respiratory rate 20/minute and unlabored, and rectal temperature was 101.8° F. He had moon facies and truncal striae. His oral mucous membranes appeared dry. His neck was supple without thyromegaly. Lung examination revealed faint scattered wheezes bilaterally. Cardiac exam was unremarkable. His abdomen was soft, with mild diffuse tenderness and no rebound tenderness. There was no hepatosplenomegaly and no masses. Bowel sounds were somewhat hyperactive but normal in quality. Rectal examination revealed no tenderness, and his stool was negative for occult blood. His extremities were notable for trace pedal edema. Neurologic exam revealed no abnormalities.

DIAGNOSTIC CLUES:

CBC:

Hematocrit: 49.5%
White blood cell count: 5,400
Platelets: 220,000

SMA:

Sodium: 129
Chloride: 95
Potassium: 5.5
HCO_3: 20
BUN: 40
Creatinine: 1.5
Glucose: 187

Urinalysis:

No cells, 1+ glucose, no ketones, no protein

Gram stain of stool:

No leukocytes seen

EKG:

Sinus tachycardia at a rate of 120/minute, normal intervals and axis, no acute changes

Chest x-ray:

No acute infiltrate, normal heart size

KUB:

Nonspecific bowel gas pattern

QUESTIONS:

1. What additional laboratory tests should be ordered?

2. What is the differential diagnosis of this patient's illness?

3. What treatment should be instituted in the Emergency Department?

4. What are possible consequences of misdiagnosis in this case?

5. What precipitating events might have led to this patient's acute illness?

ANSWERS:

1. Further evaluation of his stool is needed with stool bacterial cultures. A low-grade temperature in a patient on steroid therapy warrants blood cultures. Serum theophylline and serum cortisol levels should be drawn. Urine electrolytes and osmolality may be of limited value, since the patient is currently on diuretic therapy. A serum amylase might be useful to rule out pancreatitis, and liver function tests to rule out hepatitis or disease of the biliary tree.

2. Possibilities include viral gastroenteritis, bacterial gastrointestinal infection, theophylline toxicity, and adrenal insufficiency.

Theophylline toxicity must always be considered in the asthmatic with abdominal complaints. Early signs of toxicity include nausea, vomiting, and diarrhea as well as anxiety and tremulousness. Increasing toxicity is associated with increasing signs of central nervous instability and may result in seizures or coma. This diagnosis is a possibility but would not adequately explain his fever and electrolyte abnormalities.

The diagnosis of viral gastroenteritis or bacterial gastrointestinal infection would adequately explain his nausea, vomiting, diarrhea, abdominal pain, and fever. Gastrointestinal fluid and electrolyte losses might account for his depressed sodium, increased BUN, and increased hematocrit as well as the relatively low blood pressure in a known hypertensive. However, if this were the case, one would expect his serum potassium to be low rather than elevated.

Acute adrenal insufficiency must always be the leading diagnosis when a patient who is on chronic steroid therapy presents with abdominal symptoms, hypotension, hyponatremia, or hyperkalemia. Since serum cortisol results are not possible on an emergency basis to confirm the diagnosis, the physician must maintain a high index of suspicion. Adrenal crisis is a clinical diagnosis, not a laboratory diagnosis.

Patients with adrenal insufficiency usually present complaining of anorexia, nausea, vomiting, diarrhea, and vague abdominal pain. A history of flank pain, unexplained fever or extreme weakness may also be given. Hypotension, particularly orthostatic, is common. Mild azotemia, minimal metabolic acidosis, hyponatremia, and hyperkalemia are present in only 50% of patients. The absence of these findings does not rule out the diagnosis.

The most common cause of adrenal insufficiency is suppression of the pituitary-adrenal axis by long-term steroid therapy in pharmacologic doses. Adrenocortical destruction is a much less common cause of adrenal insufficiency, which may result from tuberculosis or fungal infection of the adrenals (a possibility in this case), autoimmune adrenalitis, sepsis (meningococcal or pneumococcal), adrenal hemorrhage secondary to anticoagulant therapy, leukemia, cancer metastatic to the adrenals (particularly lung or breast cancer), or hemochromatosis. When the adrenal gland itself is affected, the syndrome is termed primary adrenal insufficiency, or Addison's disease.

Another cause of adrenal insufficiency is deficient production of ACTH by the pituitary gland. ACTH deficiency may result from pituitary or hypothalamic destruction by tumor, surgery, head injury, or cerebrovascular accident.

3. Treatment consists of (1) glucocorticoid replacement, (2) fluid and electrolyte correction, (3) correction of hypotension, (4) correction of hyperkalemia, and (5) treatment of the underlying cause of adrenal crisis, such as trauma or infection.

In order to correct the cortisol deficit, the patient should be given an initial intravenous bolus of hydrocortisone 100 mg, followed by 100 mg every 8 hours in a continuous infusion for a total of 300 mg in the first 24 hours. Bolus doses are not an acceptable substitute for continuous infusion since effective plasma levels may not be continuously maintained. Administration of cortisone acetate 100 mg by intramuscular injection upon initial treatment and every 12 hours thereafter provides an additional source of steroid in case the intravenous infusion is inadvertently interrupted.

To correct fluid and electrolyte deficits, administer 1 L of 5% dextrose in physiological saline in the first 1 to 2 hours, followed by 1 L every 3 to 6 hours for 24 hours.

Hypotension will usually be corrected by rapid hydration with saline and replacement of glucocorticoid. Occasionally vasopressor agents are necessary, and phenylephrine hydrochloride (Neo-Synephrine) 0.25 to 0.50 mg can be given as an intravenous bolus or phenylephrine can be administered as a continuous infusion in a concentration of 4 mg/1000 cc of physiological saline at a rate of 4 μg/min.

Hyperkalemia also will usually respond to hydration and glucocorticoid therapy. If the initial serum potassium is greater than 6.5 or cardiac arrhythmias are present, 10 cc of 10% calcium chloride and one or two ampules of sodium bicarbonate can be given intravenously. Some authors also advocate administration of sodium bicarbonate if blood pH is 7.2 or less or total bicarbonate is less than 10 mEq/L.

4. Acute adrenal insufficiency is a life-threatening event. Untreated adrenal crisis may result in cardiovascular collapse and death.

5. Adrenal crisis may occur spontaneously in a patient with an extremely low cortisol output. Most patients, however, go into crisis following some stressful event in which they are unable to increase cortisol production to meet the increased requirement. Common precipitating factors include infection, trauma, surgery, general anesthesia, and excessive loss of sodium and water through sweating or diarrhea.

PEARLS:

1. The diagnosis of acute adrenal insufficiency is necessarily empiric, as there is generally no time to confirm the clinical impression.

2. Be sure to draw a serum cortisol level before therapy is instituted in order to confirm the diagnosis.

3. A normal plasma cortisol level in the context of a severe clinical stress is inappropriately low and suggestive of adrenal insufficiency. A value of less than 10 µg/dL during stress is suggestive, and less than 5 µg/dL is virtually diagnostic.

4. Hyponatremia with inappropriately high urine osmolality and sodium excretion is not always due to the syndrome of inappropriate diuretic hormone. Consider adrenocortical insufficiency, particularly in the presence of hyperkalemia, in young people, and in the absence of obvious causes.

PITFALLS:

1. Never withhold treatment if adrenal crisis is suspected. Whereas administration of hydrocortisone to a patient who is not in adrenal crisis is relatively benign, failure to treat acute adrenocortical insufficiency may be fatal.

2. A blood pressure in the normal range does not rule out adrenal crisis, particularly in a known hypertensive.

3. Do not delay therapy while awaiting results of hormone assays.

4. It is dangerous to attempt correction of the hyperkalemia of adrenal insufficiency with insulin and intravenous dextrose, as the insulin may precipitate severe hypoglycemia. The hyperkalemia will correct as the adrenal insufficiency is treated.

5. Do not let the clinical syndrome of adrenal crisis overshadow the precipitating cause. Always seek a precipitating event and treat appropriately.

REFERENCES:

Christy NP. Corticosteroid therapy and unintentional camouflage. JAMA 1988;260(14):2107-2109.

Gilliland PF. Endocrine emergencies: adrenal crisis, myxedema coma, and thyroid storm. Postgrad Med 1983;74(5):215-227.

Himathongkam T, Newmark SR, Greenfield M, Dluhy RG. Acute adrenal insufficiency. JAMA 1974;230(9):1317-1318.

Knowlton AI, Baer L. Cardiac failure in Addison's disease. Am J Med 1983;74:829-836.

Waise A, Young RJ: Pitfalls in the management of acute adrenocortical insufficiency: discussion paper. J Royal Soc Med 1989;82:741-742.

A DRIVER WITHOUT A SEAT BELT

Case 26:

A 45-year-old unrestrained male driver arrived in the Emergency Department on a spinal board with a cervical collar in place. The patient was intoxicated and could not remember any events surrounding the accident. According to the paramedics' report, the patient required extrication from the vehicle; it was also noted that the steering column of the car was deformed. Initial vital signs at the scene were blood pressure of 130/90, pulse 110/minute, and respirations 32/minute and labored.

On arrival in the Emergency Department, the patient complained of shortness of breath and right-sided chest pain. His vital signs were blood pressure of 140/100, pulse 110/minute and regular, and labored respirations at a rate of 32/minute.

Examination of the head, eyes, ears, nose, and throat revealed some bruising over the forehead but was otherwise unremarkable. The neck demonstrated a midline trachea, with no spinal tenderness or stepoff. The chest examination was notable for multiple rib fractures and paradoxical movement of the right side of the chest with decreased breath sounds over the right hemithorax. The abdomen was soft; there were decreased bowel sounds, and no rebound, guarding, or distention were noted. The extremities were without deformity, and gross motor and sensory examination revealed no deficits.

Cervical spine and pelvic films were normal. An initial arterial blood gas on 3 L/minute nasal cannula was pH 7.28, pCO_2 45, pO_2 52, and HCO_3 18.

DIAGNOSTIC CLUE:

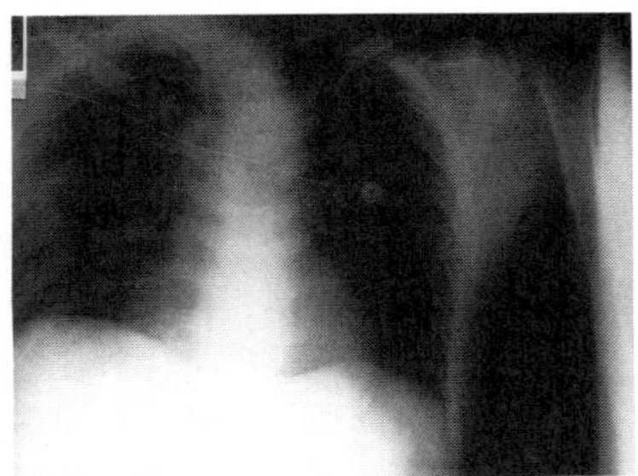

QUESTIONS:

1. What is the diagnosis and how should this patient be managed?

2. What clinical and radiographic findings suggest injury to the thoracic aorta?

3. Should the possibility of cardiac contusion be considered and how is this diagnosis made?

4. What other injuries are seen with blunt trauma to the chest?

ANSWERS:

1. In this patient, multiple rib fractures are noted as well as "paradoxical" movement of the right side of the chest cavity. Paradoxical movement of the chest means that a portion of the chest moves inward with inspiration and outward with expiration--the opposite of normal respiration. Such a combination is known as a flail chest. In order for a flail chest to occur at least two fractures in each of three adjacent ribs or costal cartilage must be present, resulting in a "free floating" segment of the chest wall. A flail may not be initially clinically apparent because of splinting.

It was previously believed that the paradoxical respirations led to impaired ventilation. Recent work has demonstrated that the underlying lung injury in the form of pulmonary contusions is responsible for the early respiratory complications. Pulmonary contusions are characterized by both intraalveolar and interstitial edema.

The x-ray findings of pulmonary contusion can vary from bilateral, diffuse patchy infiltrates to homogenous rounded consolidations. However, a key point is that consolidation will not conform to the normal segmental patterns of the lung. While the majority of patients with pulmonary contusion will show radiographic signs in the first hour, a subset of patients will not demonstrate roentgenographic findings for 4 to 6 hours. It should be noted that the size of the radiologic density does not correlate with the amount of lung damage.

The treatment and prognosis of flail chest with pulmonary contusion depends on several factors: the severity of lung injury, the nature and severity of other injuries, and the patient's age and physiologic reserve. While advances have been made in managing these patients without mechanical ventilation, it must be remembered that prevention of hypoxia is of paramount importance. The same general criteria determining the need for mechanical ventilation in other conditions leading to respiratory failure can be applied to pulmonary contusion, e.g., p_aO_2 less than 50 mm Hg, p_aCO_2 greater than 50 mm Hg, respiratory rate greater than 30 to 40/minute. It should also be kept in mind that hemopneumothorax is present in up to 70% of cases of pulmonary contusion.

2. While traumatic rupture of the aorta accounts for a large percentage of deaths immediately following a motor vehicle accident, many patients with traumatic rupture arriving at a hospital with vital signs will have few or no signs or symptoms indicating the presence of this injury. The mechanism of this injury is a sudden deceleration that leads to shearing forces developing between the mobile aortic arch and fixed descending aorta. This disruption usually occurs near the ligamentum arteriosum, which is the first point of fixation.

Those patients with aortic rupture who survive the initial insult (approximately 10%) usually have a disruption of the intima and media with an intact adventitia. If this injury is not immediately recognized, over half the patients surviving the initial injury will die within 6 hours.

Even though early diagnosis is often difficult, there are certain clues that should heighten one's suspicion of aortic rupture. Patients will most frequently complain of back or chest pain. On physical examination, dyspnea, dysphagia or hoarseness may result from compression by the expanding aorta on associated structures. Also, a "pseudocoarctation" of the aorta may be present, resulting in upper extremity hypertension with relative hypotension of the lower extremities. A thorough neurologic exam is warranted because paraplegia or paraparesis can occur as a consequence of spinal cord ischemia.

Various chest x-ray findings have been reported supporting the diagnosis of traumatic rupture of the aorta. These include (1) superior mediastinal widening, (2) an ill-defined aortic knob, (3) depression of the left mainstem bronchus, (4) tracheal deviation to the right, (5) deviation of a nasogastric tube to the right, and (6) left apical capping. Technical factors, including supine and AP views of the chest versus the normal PA view can make interpretation of mediastinal widening difficult.

While CAT scan and ultrasound are being employed with increasing frequency, a formal arch arteriogram is still the gold standard for diagnosis and the only certain means of excluding the diagnosis of traumatic aortic rupture.

3. Like aortic rupture, myocardial contusion is a diagnosis where a high index of suspicion is the key. Unlike traumatic aortic rupture, there is little agreement on any aspect of the diagnosis and management of myocardial contusion. One of the problems is that myocardial contusion can apply to injuries ranging from microscopic interstitial hemorrhage to free wall rupture.

The most common etiology for myocardial contusion is a motor vehicle accident in which a sudden deceleration or a crush injury to the chest occurs. Certain injuries and symptoms should draw attention to the potential for myocardial contusion, viz., rib fractures, sternal fractures, chest wall contusion, pulmonary contusion, anginal type chest pain, new cardiac murmurs, and any signs of cardiac tamponade. Early diagnosis of cardiac contusion is important because of its possible consequences, which range from early problems such as arrhythmia, pump failure, and conductive blocks to delayed complications such as ventricular aneurysm and cardiac rupture (immediate cardiac rupture is almost uniformly fatal).

All patients suspected of having a myocardial contusion should have supplemental oxygen provided, intravenous access established, and cardiac monitoring instituted. While the sensitivity and specificity of an EKG in diagnosing myocardial contusion is debated, most authorities agree this should be the initial study. The most frequent abnormalities are sinus tachycardia and nonspecific ST and T wave changes, but a new bundle branch block, arrhythmia, or ischemic changes may be diagnostic. Determination of cardiac enzymes, particularly CPK MB isoenzymes, should also be obtained. Again, there is much confusion in the literature concerning both positive and negative results. The CPK MB fraction can be elevated from a variety of injuries to other organs. Likewise, a normal CPK MB does not entirely rule out myocardial injury.

Much of the difficulty in assessing the various diagnostic techniques is due to the lack of a gold standard for the diagnosis. Recent enthusiasm has centered on two-dimensional echocardiography and gated radionuclide angiography. The advantages of 2-D echocardiography are that it can be done safely in either the Emergency Department or intensive care unit; it provides direct visualization of the cardiac chambers, including the presence or absence of thrombus; it allows ejection fraction to be calculated, wall motion abnormalities to be delineated, and the presence or absence of tamponade to be determined. Gated radionuclide angiography is used to assess wall motion of the heart as well as left and right ventricular ejection fractions.

In summary, any patient with an injury suggestive of myocardial contusion should have an EKG and CPK MB studies performed. If either of these is abnormal, it is prudent to obtain either 2-D echocardiography or gated radionuclide angiography. In the intervening period, these patients should be managed in a similar manner to patients with myocardial infarction, with monitoring and serial EKGs and cardiac isoenzyme determination in an intensive-care setting. Any life-threatening complications need to be addressed immediately.

4. Blunt chest trauma can occur from a variety of mechanisms--falls, explosions, contact sports, and most commonly, motor vehicle accidents. Injuries can occur to the thoracic cage, pulmonary parenchyma, tracheobronchial tree, heart, great vessels, and abdominal contents. The presentation can be as dramatic as cardiac arrest or as subtle as mild chest wall pain. Therefore, one must not only diagnose and treat the initially presenting injuries but also remain aware of pathological conditions that may become manifest with time.

Flail chest with pulmonary contusion, traumatic rupture of the aorta, and myocardial contusion have already been discussed. Other injuries that need to be addressed are rib fractures, sternal fractures, tracheobronchial injuries, and traumatic diaphragmatic hernia.

Isolated rib fractures, while not an immediately life-threatening injury, can have grave consequences, particularly in the elderly and debilitated. Because of pain, the patient splints respiration, which leads to atelectasis and possible pneumonia. Fractures usually occur at the posterior lateral angle. A chest x-ray is necessary to look for complications, i.e., pneumothorax, hemothorax, pulmonary contusion. However, complications such as pneumothorax can be delayed for up to 24 to 48 hours. While rib films are often unnecessary, trauma to the upper two ribs and lower ribs can have added significance. The upper ribs are well-protected and require significant force to cause a fracture and are associated with an increase in mortality and morbidity in trauma patients. Fractures of ribs 9 to 12 should alert the clinician to possible intraabdominal or renal injury.

Mild to moderate pain from a simple rib fracture can usually be managed with analgesia or intercostal nerve block. It is prudent to hospitalize patients with more than two rib fractures, particularly elderly patients or patients with underlying lung disease.

Sternal fractures also imply severe chest trauma and warrant a careful search for other injuries, particularly myocardial contusion and aortic disruption. Sternal fractures are best seen on a lateral view of the chest.

Tracheobronchial injuries, while frequently fatal, are often missed initially. The clinical presentation is variable and depends on the degree of communication between the trachea and/or bronchus with the pleura, ranging from massive subcutaneous air and mediastinal emphysema to a persistent pneumothorax. Bronchoscopy is required to make the diagnosis.

Traumatic asphyxia can also occur from blunt trauma to the chest. The clinical picture is often dramatic, with subconjunctival hemorrhage and petechiae and vascular engorgement, edema, and cyanosis of the head, neck, and upper extremities. Management is the same as for all chest trauma patients.

Another elusive injury with blunt trauma to the chest is diaphragmatic rupture. Rarely is this an isolated injury, and it is frequently overshadowed by accompanying injuries. The location of the rupture is most commonly on the left side of the chest in the retrosternal portion of the diaphragm. Recognition of this injury is essential to prevent herniation of the abdominal contents into the chest cavity, which will compress the lungs, impairing ventilation and leading to hypoxia. Early recognition depends on a high degree of suspicion, heightened when the chest x-ray appears to have either an elevated left diaphragm or a loculated pneumothorax. Early management should involve placement of a nasogastric tube and arrangement should be made for either CAT scan or contrast radiography to confirm the diagnosis.

PEARLS:

1. Thoracic trauma is the second leading cause of death and disability in trauma patients (head trauma is number one).

2. A persistent air leak with a pneumothorax is indicative of (1) improper position of the chest tube (make sure all the holes of the tube are in the pleural cavity) or (2) bronchial

occlusion or laceration (bronchopleural fistula). If the chest tube system is functioning properly, emergency bronchoscopy is indicated.

3. Fractures of the lower left ribs are associated with splenic trauma in up to 20% of cases, and hepatic trauma is seen in up to 10% of fractures of ribs 9 to 12 on the right.

4. The incidence of rupture of the aorta in persons thrown from a vehicle is more than twice that of victims not ejected.

5. It usually takes 250 to 400 cc of fluid to blunt the costophrenic angles in an upright chest x-ray.

PITFALLS:

1. Restoration of adequate circulating volume is of paramount importance. This should not be sacrificed to "keep the patient on the dry side." Adequate volume resuscitation, not overresuscitation, is the goal.

2. Chest x-rays often underestimate the degree of pulmonary insult. The alveolar-arterial gradient is a more sensitive indicator of pulmonary parenchymal damage.

3. Don't apply rib belts, tape the chest wall, or apply sand bags to the chest for rib fractures. These not only offer no help but are harmful in that they limit chest wall expansion in uninjured segments of the chest wall leading to atelectasis.

4. What appears to be a pneumothorax on the left side of the chest could be a ruptured diaphragm with a concomitant air-filled viscus in the chest. Inadvertent placement of a chest tube into this structure could be disastrous. This is why it is necessary to confirm with a finger the presence of a free pleural cavity before insertion of a tube.

REFERENCES:

Hossack KF, Movena CA, VanWay CW, Burdick DC. Frequency of cardiac contusion with nonpenetrating chest trauma. Am J Cardio 1988;61:391-394.

Marnocha KE, Maglinte DT. Blunt chest trauma and aortic rupture: reliability of chest radiograph findings. Ann Emerg Med 1985;14:644-649.

Richardson JD, Adams L, Flint LM. Selective management of flail chest and pulmonary contusion. Ann Surg 1982;196:481-487.

Tenzer ML. The spectrum of myocardial contusion: a review. J Trauma 1985;25:620-627.

Trunkey DD. Torso trauma. Curr Prob Surg 1987;24:209-265.

Wiot JF. The radiologic manifestations of blunt chest trauma. JAMA 1975;231:500-506.

A TEENAGER WITH PELVIC PAIN

Case 27:

A 19-year-old female presented to the Emergency Department complaining of abdominal pain for the past 2 days. She stated she was in her usual state of health until 2 days earlier when she noted a dull ache in her right lower abdomen. The ache was initially intermittent but gradually became constant and increased in intensity, with minimal improvement in response to ibuprofen. Several hours prior to her coming to the Emergency Department, the pain became severe and spread throughout her lower abdomen.

She denied any dysuria, hematuria, constipation, diarrhea, melena, hematochezia, vaginal discharge, or vaginal bleeding. She was a sexually active female who had never been pregnant and used condoms and contraceptive foam as her method of birth control. Her last menstrual period was 6 weeks earlier, but the patient stated that her menses were generally irregular and normally ranged from 4 to 6 weeks between menses. She stated she had one episode of pelvic inflammatory disease 2 years earlier and had been treated with antibiotics as an outpatient.

On physical examination, the patient was a thin female in moderate distress. Her blood pressure was 90/50 both standing and supine, and her pulse was 90/minute both standing and supine. Her respiratory rate was 20/minute and regular, and her rectal temperature was 100.4° F. Exam of her head, eyes, ears, nose, and throat was unremarkable. Her lungs were clear, and her heart sounds were normal without any murmurs or gallops.

Her abdomen was soft but the patient exhibited much guarding with localized rebound tenderness over both lower quadrants. There was no hepatosplenomegaly or masses palpable. Bowel sounds were present, but hypoactive. Pelvic examination revealed a scant brown vaginal discharge. Her cervix was notable for marked motion tenderness, and both her uterus and adnexae were diffusely tender with increased tenderness over the right adnexa. Examination was limited due to much guarding on the part of the patient. Rectal examination revealed brown stool which was negative for occult blood and notable only for mild diffuse tenderness on digital examination.

DIAGNOSTIC CLUES:

Hematocrit: 35%
Serum white blood cell count: 12,000
Platelets: Normal
PT/PTT: Normal
Culdocentesis: No fluid aspirated
Urine pregnancy test: Negative

QUESTIONS:

1. What is the differential diagnosis of this patient's problem?
2. What information is provided by the culdocentesis?
3. What further diagnostic tests should the physician order?
4. What treatment should be instituted in the Emergency Department?
5. Describe possible sequelae in this case.

ANSWERS:

1. A young woman with right lower quadrant pain presents a diagnostic challenge. Possibilities include gynecologic disorders such as ectopic pregnancy, ruptured ovarian cyst, ovarian torsion, and pelvic inflammatory disease as well as acute appendicitis. Of greatest concern in this case is the possibility of a tubal pregnancy, as a ruptured tubal pregnancy is a gynecologic emergency. A young woman with a history of late menses and severe pelvic pain must be presumed to have a tubal pregnancy until proven otherwise. Risk factors for ectopic pregnancy include previous ectopic pregnancy, current intrauterine device use, prior fallopian tube surgery, previous pelvic inflammatory disease, pelvic surgery, use of high progesterone oral contraceptives, and a prior history of infertility. Abdominal pain is the most common symptom, followed by amenorrhea or vaginal bleeding, nausea, vomiting, syncope, and dizziness. Referred shoulder pain following the onset of abdominal pain is characteristic of intraperitoneal bleeding.

2. A positive result on culdocentesis for ruptured ectopic pregnancy is usually considered to be more than 2 cc of nonclotting blood. If the aspirate clots or the hematocrit is <15%, the test is considered negative. Aspiration of pus is usually indicative of infection, typically pelvic inflammatory disease. Serosanguineous fluid is suggestive of a ruptured ovarian cyst. Clear fluid or no fluid on aspiration are considered to be negative, but these results must be interpreted with caution.

3. Although culdocentesis was previously considered the gold standard for the diagnosis of a ruptured tubal pregnancy, in recent years ultrasonography, and particularly transvaginal ultrasonography, in combination with a sensitive serum human chorionic gonadotropin assay have become the primary diagnostic modalities. A provisional diagnosis of ectopic pregnancy may be established if the uterus is empty on transabdominal sonography and the HCG value is greater than 6500 mIU/cc.

4. Treatment in the Emergency Department should begin with placing a large-bore intravenous catheter and supporting blood pressure if there is any instability. A serum pregnancy test should be ordered immediately and sonography ordered, provided there will be no significant delay. If a significant delay is anticipated, emergency laparoscopy or laparotomy is indicated. Laparoscopy has gained a great deal of popularity in recent years, allowing both increased accuracy in diagnosis for a variety of acute intraabdominal complaints as well as another surgical option, with both appendectomy and cholecystectomy now being performed via laparoscope.

5. An untreated ruptured ectopic pregnancy carries a significant morbidity and mortality. The incidence of ectopic pregnancy has quadrupled since 1970; during this same period,

there was a sevenfold decrease in maternal mortality, which has been attributed to technologic advances in diagnosis. However, in over half of reported maternal deaths from ruptured ectopic pregnancy, the patient was seen during the preceding 48 hours by a physician. A high index of suspicion combined with appropriate use of laboratory and ultrasound technologies is essential for the diagnosis not to be missed.

Patients who are treated appropriately for an ectopic pregnancy may have either salpingotomy or salpingectomy, and their overall fertility remains poor. Only 30% of women treated with salpingectomy subsequently experience term pregnancy. With conservative surgical treatment, future fertility is preserved in 50 to 60% of women with ectopic pregnancies.

PEARLS:

1. A negative or nondiagnostic culdocentesis does not exclude the possibility of tubal rupture and should not give you a false sense of security. In contradistinction, a positive tap does not imply tubal rupture and should not constitute an excuse for emergency laparotomy in a hemodynamically stable patient.

2. In ectopic pregnancy, the uterus is usually normal in size, but may be enlarged from deciduation, accumulation of blood, or multiparity.

3. Contralateral tenderness may be due to a corpus luteum cyst, which occurs opposite an ectopic pregnancy in up to 15% of cases.

4. Cul-de-sac fullness may represent either clotted blood or an enlarged adnexa positioned dependently in the pelvis.

5. Cervical motion may evoke adnexal tenderness in ectopic pregnancy.

PITFALLS:

1. Although vaginal bleeding due to ectopic pregnancy is not as great as that associated with spontaneous abortion, heavy bleeding should not be viewed as incompatible with ectopic pregnancy.

2. Significant orthostatic changes usually do not occur in otherwise healthy women until 10 to 15% of the blood volume is lost.

3. An adnexal mass is palpable in approximately 50% of cases. The absence of an adnexal mass does not exclude the diagnosis of ectopic pregnancy.

4. Hypotension in young females is difficult to define because many young women normally have blood pressures in the low-normal range compared with older or male patients.

5. Studies have shown that tachycardia is an unreliable indicator of shock in young women with ruptured ectopic pregnancies.

6. Do not interpret a decidual reaction of the uterus (seen with ectopic pregnancy) as a developing intrauterine pregnancy on ultrasound.

REFERENCES:

Leach RE, Ory SJ. Management of ectopic pregnancy. Am Fam Physician 1990;41(4):1215-1222.

Ory SJ. Ectopic pregnancy: current evaluation and treatment. Mayo Clin Proc 1989;64(7):874-877.

Schwab RA. Ultrasound versus culdocentesis in the evaluation of early and late ectopic pregnancy. Ann Emerg Med 1988;17(8):801-803.

Snyder HS. Lack of a tachycardic response to hypotension with ruptured ectopic pregnancy. Am J Emerg Med 1990;8(1):23-26.

Vermesh M, Graczykowski JW, Sauer MV. Reevaluation of the role of culdocentesis in the management of ectopic pregnancy. Am J Obstet Gynecol 1990;162(2):411-413.

A SECRETARY WITH A HEADACHE

Case 28:

A 52-year-old medical secretary and hospital employee came to the Emergency Department complaining of a severe headache for a half hour. She had been in her usual state of health, typing at her office desk, when she noted the sudden onset of a severe bilateral headache which radiated down her neck to her upper back. She became nauseated, vomited once, and left her desk to walk to the Emergency Department with a friend. She denied loss of consciousness of any other acute neurologic symptoms.

The patient stated she had a long-standing history of migraine headaches, usually associated with menses, and typically consisting of a unilateral headache which was often associated with nausea and dizziness, and less commonly associated with vomiting or scotomata. The headaches occurred once every 2 to 3 months and were usually relieved by two tablets of Fioricet and bedrest. She stated her current headache was similar in quality to her usual migraines, but "10 times" more severe. She stated she had a similar headache and backache 1 week earlier while typing, which she treated by going home, taking two tablets of Fioricet, and sleeping for 6 hours. She denied any other significant medical history, and stated she was taking no other medications.

On physical examination, she was a somewhat distraught middle-aged female, complaining of a headache. Her blood pressure was 160/90, her pulse was 90/minute and regular, her respiratory rate was 12/minute, and a rectal temperature was 100.8° F. Examination of her lungs, heart, and abdomen was unremarkable. Ophthalmoscopic examination was difficult, but both optic disks appeared flat. Her neck was supple, but the patient complained of severe pain radiating down her back upon anteroflexion. On neurologic examination, her cranial nerves were intact and no motor or sensory deficits were elicited. Her cerebellar examination and gait were normal. Her deep tendon reflexes were normal and bilaterally symmetrical, with no pathologic reflexes elicited. She was alert and oriented, with normal cognition and speech.

DIAGNOSTIC CLUES:

SMA:

Sodium: 140
Chloride: 101
Potassium: 3.7
Bicarbonate: 25
BUN: 22
Creatinine: 1.4
Glucose: 122

CBC:

Hematocrit: 39%
White blood cell count: 12,000 with a normal differential count
Platelets: 222,000

Protime: 12

EKG:

Sinus tachycardia at a rate of 100/minute, with nonspecific ST segment and T wave changes

Head CAT: Unremarkable

Lumbar puncture: Xanthochromic fluid

QUESTIONS:

1. What is the diagnosis?

2. What factors placed this patient at increased risk for this condition?

3. Of what significance is her previous history of headache?

4. What other physical findings might this patient have presented with?

5. Should further diagnostic testing be performed?

6. What treatment should be instituted?

7. What is this patient's prognosis?

ANSWERS:

1. This patient's clinical presentation is strongly suggestive of a subarachnoid hemorrhage. Subarachnoid hemorrhage may be separated into traumatic and spontaneous types. Spontaneous subarachnoid hemorrhage can be further subdivided into primary and secondary types.

I. Traumatic

II. Spontaneous

A. Primary (directly within subarachnoid space)
1. Congenital blood vessel abnormalities (aneurysm or arteriovenous malformation)
2. Cryptogenic

B. Secondary (extension of a parenchymal hemorrhage)
1. Hypertension
2. Blood dyscrasia or anticoagulant therapy
3. Neoplasm
4. Arteriopathy

Intracranial aneurysms are the most common cause of subarachnoid hemorrhage. Aneurysms may be classified as arteriosclerotic (fusiform), mycotic (bacterial), saccular (berry), or traumatic. Most intracranial aneurysms are saccular and arise from a bifurcation of vessels that form the circle of Willis. Saccular aneurysms usually are not congenital but develop and enlarge in adult life. Acquired factors such as arteriosclerosis and hypertension may contribute to their development or enlargement.

Arteriovenous malformations are congenital vascular anomalies in which the normal capillary bed connecting the arterial and venous systems has failed to develop. Consequently, vessels feeding the malformation become dilated and transmit blood under arterial pressure into the venous system. Arteriovenous malformations are much less common than aneurysms. The majority of arteriovenous malformation hemorrhages occur before age 40, while aneurysmal hemorrhages are uncommon before age 20.

2. Subarachnoid hemorrhage accounts for about 10% of all strokes in the United States. Risk factors include aging, female gender, hypertension, use of oral contraceptives, cigarette smoking, and alcohol consumption. Intracranial aneurysms, the most common cause of subarachnoid hemorrhage, occur in all age groups and are more common in women than in men by a 3:2 ratio. The peak incidence of rupture is between the ages of 40 and 60.

Associated medical conditions in patients with aneurysmal subarachnoid hemorrhage include coarctation of the aorta, polycystic kidney disease, connective tissue disorders, and fibromuscular dysplasia. In up to 20% of cases of subarachnoid hemorrhage, no cause can be determined.

3. Her previous history of migraines is probably not related to the subarachnoid hemorrhage. However, the headache she described 1 week earlier is highly significant. Up to 40% of patients with a ruptured aneurysm have some type of warning prior to catastrophic bleeding. This "warning leak" or "sentinel headache" may be very mild or relatively severe and should be suspected in any patient who develops new and severe headaches; it occurs without a depressed level of consciousness.

Pain is usually described in the suboccipital region, which corresponds with the blood circulating through the subarachnoid space and the basal regions of the brain. Subsequent hemolysis may lead to irritation and inflammation of the meninges, producing nuchal rigidity and pain. If the sentinel headache is relatively mild, however, the patient is not likely to seek medical attention.

4. The classic symptom is "the worst headache of my life," an event which usually heralds the rupture. Patients often have associated symptoms, including nausea and vomiting, transient loss of consciousness, confusion or lethargy, frank coma, seizure activity, and neck pain or stiffness. Aneurysms may also present with focal neurologic findings, such as an isolated third nerve palsy with or without pupillary sparing.

Early damage usually reflects the brain's intolerance of the initial hemorrhage and often occurs before the patient receives medical attention. Immediate problems may include fatal cardiac arrhythmia, intracerebral or intraventricular extension of the hemorrhage, or acute hydrocephalus. Late problems include rebleeding, delayed hydrocephalus, and delayed arterial vasospasm, which may depend not only on the amount of blood in the subarachnoid space but also on the type of treatment used.

5. If the head CAT scan demonstrates a subarachnoid hemorrhage, no additional diagnostic studies are required in the Emergency Department. If the head CAT scan is nondiagnostic, emergency lumbar puncture should be performed, provided there is no evidence of mass lesion or obstructive hydrocephalus. Blood within the spinal fluid should be present in virtually all cases of acute subarachnoid hemorrhage. Xanthochromia usually develops 4 to 6 hours after the initial hemorrhage and persists for several days. Cerebral angiography is not usually a part of the Emergency Department evaluation and its timing is generally determined by the neurosurgeon.

6. Stuporous or comatose patients should be placed on assisted ventilation to ensure adequate oxygenation. Hyperventilation is used to control elevated intracranial pressure. Blood pressure must be monitored and controlled to maintain adequate cerebral perfusion while avoiding pressure surges and excessive elevations. An effort should be made to keep the diastolic pressure under 100 mg Hg when hypertension accompanies subarachnoid bleeding. Anticonvulsants are used to prevent seizures. Corticosteroids are administered to try to decrease cerebral edema. Although controversial, antifibrinolytic therapy may be used to present rebleeding. Nimodipine, a calcium channel blocker, has been shown to reduce the occurrence of ischemic neurologic deficits associated with delayed vasospasm and may be indicated.

All patients with subarachnoid hemorrhage will require admission to an intensive care unit and emergency neurosurgical consultation. The neurosurgeon will determine the need for evacuation of acute intracerebral hematoma or intraventricular drainage procedures and will determine the timing for angiography and intracerebral aneurysm clipping. The optimal timing of definitive remains controversial. Recent studies have demonstrated improved neurologic outcome with early surgical intervention within 72 hours after the initial bleed, particularly in patients with low grades of surgical risk.

7. The ultimate surgical outcome is usually related to the patient's clinical grade at the time of surgery. The following grading system is commonly utilized:

Grade	Criteria
0	Unruptured aneurysm
I	Minimal headache or nuchal rigidity, or asymptomatic
Ia	Fixed neurologic deficit without acute meningeal or brain reaction
II	Absence of neurologic deficit with moderate to severe headache or nuchal rigidity
III	Drowsiness, confusion, or mild focal deficit
IV	Stupor, moderate or severe hemiparesis, possible early decerebrate rigidity, or vegetative disturbances
V	Deep coma, decerebrate rigidity, or moribund state

Patients in grades 0 through II generally have an excellent chance of surviving surgery with good neurologic outcomes. Grade V patients, who have had severe hemorrhages, are generally not subjected to surgical intervention unless large, life-threatening clots are evident. In general, early surgical intervention is indicated in patients of lower grades, while there is a tendency to delay surgery in patients of higher clinical grade.

PEARLS:

1. Up to 40% of patient with a ruptured aneurysm have some type of warning prior to catastrophic bleeding. This "warning leak" should be suspected in any patient who develops new and severe headaches.

2. Following subarachnoid hemorrhage, autonomic disturbances are common due to increased intracranial pressure or irritative effects of blood near vital control centers. These include ST segment changes on EKG, changes in blood pressure, vomiting, fever, and elevation of the white blood cell count.

3. Subhyaloid or preretinal hemorrhages are small, smooth, round hemorrhages usually located near the optic nerve head and believed to be virtually diagnostic of subarachnoid hemorrhage.

PITFALLS:

1. One recent survey found that the most common cause of an isolated third nerve palsy with or without pupillary sparing was a cerebral aneurysm, not diabetes.

2. If a "sentinel" or "warning" hemorrhage goes unrecognized, subsequent hemorrhage is often quite severe and carries a much higher risk of major morbidity or mortality.

3. A small subarachnoid bleed may be missed on CAT scan. A lumbar puncture is indicated following normal head CAT scan if a diagnosis of subarachnoid hemorrhage is likely.

REFERENCES:

Day AL, Salcman M. Subarachnoid hemorrhage. Am Fam Physician 1989;40(1):95-105.

Fontanarosa PB. Recognition of subarachnoid hemorrhage. Ann Emerg Med 1989;18(11):1199-1205.

Longstreth WT Jr, Koepsell TD, Yerby MS, van Belle G. Risk factors for subarachnoid hemorrhage. Stroke 1985;16(3):377-385.

Marton KI, Gean AD. The spinal tap: a new look at an old test. Ann Intern Med 1986;104(6):840-848.

Wong MC, Haley EC Jr. Calcium antagonists: stroke therapy coming of age. Stroke 1990;21(3):494-501.

ACUTE DYSPNEA AND CHEST PAIN

Case 29:

A 26-year-old construction worker was brought in by ambulance. He was driving his car when he felt the sudden onset of severe retrosternal chest pain and acute difficulty breathing. He was unable to continue driving and pulled off the road. A passerby called an ambulance.

He had no past medical history of asthma, pneumonia, or lung or heart disease, and denied any recent trauma. He was on no medications and denied any allergies. He smoked one pack per day for 5 years, drank a six-pack of beer weekly, and denied any recreational drug use. His family history was negative for cardiovascular disease.

He was a muscular young man in acute respiratory distress, gasping for air. His blood pressure was 140/80, his pulse was 100/minute, his respiratory rate was 35/minute and shallow, and his temperature was 98.0° F. His coloring was pale, but not cyanotic. His breath sounds were distant bilaterally, without wheezing, rales, or rhonchi. His heart sounds revealed a normal S1 and S2 without murmurs, gallops, or rubs. His abdominal exam was unremarkable. His extremities showed no clubbing or edema.

DIAGNOSTIC CLUES:

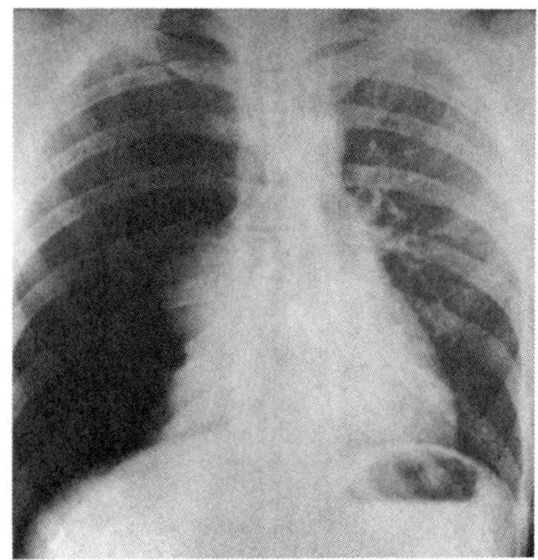

QUESTIONS:

1. What are the diagnostic possibilities?

2. What essential pieces of information did the physician neglect to note on physical examination?

3. What factors may predispose to this problem?

4. What is the appropriate acute therapy?

5. What long-term therapy is available?

ANSWERS:

1. Acute onset of chest pain and dyspnea in a young male is highly suggestive of spontaneous pneumothorax. Other diagnostic possibilities include acute myocardial infarction, new onset crescendo angina, anaphylactic reaction, new onset asthma with severe bronchospasm, acute cardiac arrhythmia such as atrial fibrillation, cardiac tamponade, acute aortic dissection, or acute pulmonary embolus.

These diagnostic possibilities must be assessed rapidly and accurately, as these disorders are potentially life-threatening. Acute evaluation of this patient begins with assessment of vital signs and physical examination of the heart and lungs. An electrocardiogram should be obtained immediately. A baseline arterial blood gas should be drawn and oxygen supplementation should be provided. A chest x-ray should be obtained emergently if at all possible.

In this case the chest x-ray provides the diagnosis of tension pneumothorax. Radiographic findings in tension pneumothorax include hyperlucency of the lung field in the area of collapse and shift of mediastinal structures and the trachea to the unaffected side, due to increased pleural pressure on the side of the collapse.

When a pneumothorax is suspected, a radiograph should be obtained with the patient in the erect position or the decubitus position with the involved side up. End-expiratory films are often preferred because lung volume is then smallest and the pneumothorax is most easily visualized.

Pneumothorax appears on x-ray as a very thin, sharp, white line between air in the lung and pleural space. Pneumothorax can be simulated by a skin fold, but can be differentiated by the following criteria:

a. Vascular shadows extend peripheral to a skin fold
b. A skin fold typically extends peripheral to the rib shadows
c. Skin folds are frequently multiple and bilateral
d. Skin folds usually produce a zone of gradually changing optical density medial to the interface

If doubt remains regarding the radiographic interpretation, additional decubitus or erect views should be obtained.

2. The physician did not record the examination of the neck. Of particular importance is the position of the trachea, a critical point in evaluation of a possible spontaneous pneumothorax. Tracheal deviation toward the unaffected lung is common in tension pneumothorax. In addition, there is no mention of the presence or absence of neck vein

distention, commonly seen in both pneumothorax and acute cardiac disorders.

On the lung exam, auscultation was performed without specific findings. The physician should have quickly augmented this unremarkable examination with percussion (looking for increased resonance on the side of collapse) and evaluation of tactile fremitus (decreased on the side of collapse). In addition, the chest wall may show overexpansion on the side of the pneumothorax.

3. Spontaneous pneumothorax can be classified by etiology, physiology, or magnitude.

   a. Etiology
      Spontaneous
      Traumatic
      Iatrogenic

   b. Physiology
      Open
      Closed
      Tension

   c. Magnitude (percentage of collapsed lung)

Spontaneous pneumothorax occurs five times more often in males. Approximately 60% of patients with spontaneous pneumothorax will eventually have a recurrence on the ipsilateral side; 15% will have one on the contralateral side. Most spontaneous pneumothoraces are probably due to the spontaneous rupture of subpleural blebs.

Asthmatics may develop mediastinal emphysema, which can then track into the pleural cavity. Other causes of spontaneous pneumothorax include infections (pneumonia, tuberculosis, fungal infections, lung abscesses), some connective tissue disorders (e.g., scleroderma), connective tissue defects (e.g., Marfan's syndrome), neoplasms (either primary or metastatic), sarcoidosis, fibrotic lung disease, and endometriosis.

Surprisingly, traumatic pneumothorax can be caused by a vigorous cough or exertion involving the Valsalva maneuver. Any injury causing perforation of the chest wall, trachea, or bronchial tree or the barometric pressure variations experienced by divers can result in collapse.

Iatrogenic pneumothorax is most often caused by procedures such as central line insertion, endotracheal intubation, bronchoscopy, or thoracentesis or by the use of mechanical ventilators.

4. Acute therapy depends on the type and magnitude of the pneumothorax. The two main problems with tension pneumothorax are hypoxia and hypotension. Tension pneumothorax is a complication of a simple pneumothorax which occurs when, for some reason, the injury creates a one-way ball-valve effect so that air enters the pleural space with each inspiration but is unable to escape. Thus pressure in the pleural space builds with each breath.

In tension pneumothorax, hypotension may be the result of increased intrathoracic pressure with decreased venous return, or shifting of mediastinal structures with kinking of major vessels. Emergency treatment involves the insertion of a needle or intravenous catheter in the second intercostal space in the midclavicular line directly into the pleural cavity to relieve the pressure. More definitive treatment requires chest tube thoracostomy (usually inserted in the fifth intercostal space in the midaxillary line).

Emergency treatment of an open pneumothorax consists of placing an airtight dressing (e.g., petrolatum gauze) directly over the open chest wound and, it is hoped, converting an open pneumothorax to a closed one. A chest tube can be inserted later. Definitive treatment is surgical.

The acute treatment of closed pneumothorax varies, depending on the magnitude of the pneumothorax, presence of other disorders, and history of previous pneumothorax. In healthy patients who are tolerating a pneumothorax whose magnitude is roughly 25% or less, hospitalization for bedrest and serial chest films may be sufficient. About 1% of normal lung volume will be reabsorbed daily. Theoretically, nasal oxygen is of value, because oxygen administration will cause a decrease in alveolar nitrogen concentration and the "room air" in the pleural cavity (which is 80% nitrogen) will travel down the nitrogen concentration gradient to the alveolar space.

Tube thoracostomy is generally the treatment of choice in patients with pulmonary or other serious disease, pneumothoraces greater than 25%, recurrent pneumothorax, and pneumothoraces associated with trauma.

5. Pleurodesis, the adherence of visceral to parietal pleura, is available as prophylactic therapy to prevent recurrent pneumothorax. Simple tube thoracostomy will cause local pleural irritation with subsequent adhesion. Sometimes irritating substances, such as tetracycline, are instilled directly into the pleural cavity to cause adhesions. However, this method is generally quite painful and sometimes ineffective. The most effective method of pleurodesis is thoracotomy with direct scraping of the parietal pleura with gauze; however, this incurs the risks of a surgical procedure.

PEARLS:

1. Subcutaneous emphysema may be apparent on examination as a "crackling cellophane" sensation on palpation of the skin overlying the abdomen, chest, and neck.

2. Mediastinal emphysema may be apparent as a crackling sound heard on auscultation, coordinated with the heartbeat ("Hamman's crunch").

3. Placement of a large-bore needle into the second intercostal space at the midclavicular line over the pneumothorax may be both diagnostic and therapeutic.

PITFALLS:

1. Chest x-ray will confirm the diagnosis, but treatment should not be delayed awaiting x-ray if the patient is acutely ill and the diagnosis is apparent.

2. Due to ventilation/perfusion mismatching, patients with collapse will initially demonstrate some degree of hypoxia on blood gas. After several hours, perfusion of the affected lung decreases, with resultant improvement in ventilation/perfusion ratios and some resolution of hypoxia.

3. Do not overtreat. A stable patient with a closed pneumothorax of less than 25% magnitude does not require emergent tube thoracostomy. However, patients with even a small pneumothorax being placed on ventilators will require tube placement.

4. Do not forget to rule out pneumothoax in a patient abusing inhalational dugs who presents with chest pain.

REFERENCES:

Lesur O, Delorme N, Fromaget JM, et al. Computed tomography in the etiologic assessment of idiopathic spontaneous pneumothorax. Chest 1990;98(2):341-347.

Mann H. Common errors in evaluating chest radiographs. Postgrad Med 1990;87(1):275-278, 281-212.

O'Rourke JP, Yee ES. Civilian spontaneous pneumothorax. Treatment options and long-term results. Chest 1989;96(6):1302-1306.

Westaby S, Brayley N. ABC of major trauma. Thoracic trauma--I. Br Med J 1990;300(6740):1639-1643.

Wong DH, Stemmer EA, Gordon I. Acute massive airleak and pressure support ventilation. Crit Care Med 1990;18(1):114-115.

RECTAL PAIN IN A MIDDLE AGED MAN

Case 30:

A 45-year-old male presented to the Emergency Department complaining of acute onset of rectal pain accompanied by rectal bleeding. He stated that the pain began in the morning, when he attempted a bowel movement. He was unable to have a bowel movement and noted bright red blood on the toilet paper. The previous day he had a normal bowel movement without pain, bleeding, or discomfort. He denied nausea, vomiting, or urinary symptoms, although he did note an abdominal "fullness."

The patient gave a history of hemorrhoids, with rare rectal spotting and swelling with pain. He stated he was a social drinker, adding that he got "smashed" the night before. He denied use of illicit drugs. His past medical history was otherwise unremarkable and he had no history of surgery.

Vital signs revealed a pulse of 84/minute and regular, blood pressure of 134/88 both sitting and supine, respiratory rate of 14/minute, and temperature 99.2° F orally. Physical examination was unremarkable except for "active" bowel sounds and a mildly distended abdomen. Otherwise the abdomen was nontender without rebound or guarding. Rectal examination revealed nonthrombosed external hemorrhoids which were not actively bleeding. A digital exam revealed adequate rectal tone with scant red blood mixed with mucus. No masses were palpated.

DIAGNOSTIC CLUE:

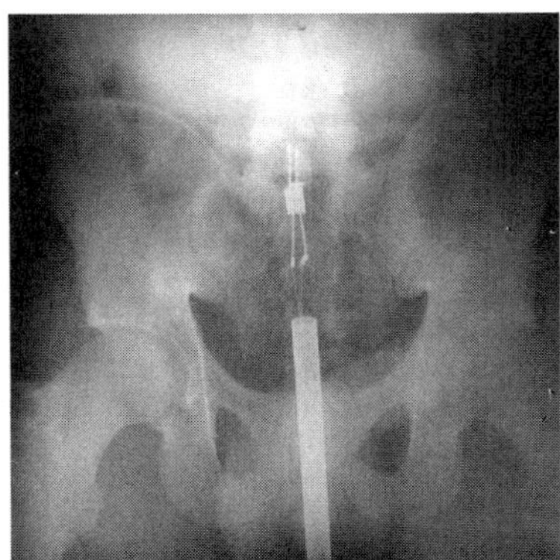

QUESTIONS:

1. What is the differential diagnosis of rectal pain?
2. What are the diagnostic steps in the evaluation of a patient with rectal pain?
3. How should this man's problem be treated?
4. What are possible complications?

ANSWERS:

1. While anorectal disorders are common, patients are often reluctant to discuss them with their physicians. This reluctance is compounded in the impersonal setting of the Emergency Department. It is often only after home remedies have failed that patients with an anorectal complaint will find their way to the Emergency Department.

Anorectal disorders usually present as one of four complaints: (1) anorectal pain with bleeding, (2) anorectal pain without bleeding, (3) painless rectal bleeding, and (4) masses without pain or bleeding. The patient in question presented with rectal pain and bleeding.

To properly understand rectal pain, a basic understanding of the fundamental anatomy of this area is essential. The true anal canal consists of stratified squamous epithelium which is somatically innervated and therefore pain sensitive. Above this stratified squamous epithelium is moist red columnar epithelium, which is relatively pain insensitive. The dentate, or pectinate line, is the demarcation between these two different cell types. The significance of the difference in cell structure is illustrated by the fact that external hemorrhoids originate below the pectinate line and becomes exquisitely tender when thrombosed. Internal hemorrhoids from above the pectinate line are covered by columnar epithelium and usually do not become as painful.

What could cause a rapid onset of rectal pain and bleeding? The most likely etiologies are a thrombosed external hemorrhoid, anal fissure, infection, or trauma. An acute external thrombosed hemorrhoid would be evident on visual inspection of the anus as a tense, dark blue nodule on the anal verge. An anal fissure is simply a "tear" in the anal tissue with its exact etiology unknown. Anal fissures usually present as a tearing or burning pain after defecation, but can cause intense spasm of the anal sphincter inhibiting bowel movements.

Infection can cause rectal pain in the form of either an abscess or a proctitis. An anorectal abscess usually results from blockage of the ducts of the anal glands and will vary in degree and quality of pain, depending on location, i.e., perianal, ischiorectal, submucosal, or supralevator. The etiologic agent in infectious proctitis depends on the sexual practices of the individual. Nonvenereal infections include Salmonella, Shigella, Campylobacter and Yersinia. Sexually transmitted pathogens such as Neisseria gonorrhoea, herpes simplex, Chlamydia trachomatis,and syphilis are more common in homosexual men and in women who engage in anal coitus.

Finally, various forms of sexual practices, namely insertion of foreign objects and fist fornication, whether voluntary or involuntary, can result in rectal pain with bleeding secondary to tearing of the mucosa.

2. After carefully inspecting the perianal region, looking for lesions, redness, or swelling, carefully palpate the region for induration, fluctuance, or tenderness. Since the anal

sphincter reflexly contracts when touched, apply gentle steady pressure with a lubricated gloved finger. The axis of the anal canal is in line with the patient's umbilicus. Remember that the canal is quite short.

After assessing rectal tone, note the presence and character of stool in the rectum, testing for occult blood. Also palpate the prostate and feel for any masses. Valuable adjuncts that can be employed in the Emergency Department are the anoscope and sigmoidoscope. An anoscope commands little skill and does not require any bowel preparation. The anoscope is directed anteriorly towards the midline and once fully inserted the obturator is removed. While withdrawing the anoscope the anal canal is inspected for internal hemorrhoids, polyps, etc.

Requiring slightly more skill but extremely valuable in the workup of rectal complaints is the rigid sigmoidoscope. When used at the bedside, the patient is placed in the left lateral Sim's position with the thighs flexed, the upper one more than the lower. The sigmoidoscope is inserted into the anus and initially directed toward the umbilicus. Once the sigmoidoscope is inserted approximately 4 cm, the obturator is removed and further advancement is only under direct visualization. At the 10- to 12-cm mark, the rectosigmoid junction is encountered. This is where the bowel sharply angulates anterior and to the left. Care must be taken when compromising this curve to not force the sigmoidoscope as perforation of the bowel can easily result. The sigmoidoscope should never be forced past the point of resistance. Periodic insufflation of the rectum and sigmoid will assist visualization. Sigmoidoscopy can be invaluable in locating the source of bleeding.

Pelvic roentgenograms should be obtain if the possibility of a foreign body or gas-forming infection exists. In our patient, a sigmoidoscope examination revealed a foreign object approximately 10 cm from the anus at the rectosigmoid junction. X-rays were subsequently obtained to confirm the position of the object. On repeat questioning, the patient sheepishly recalled one of his friends "showing off" a vibrator he had purchased. The patient stated that after a few drinks he grew curious about it. He further admitted repeated efforts were unsuccessful in retrieving the object.

Types of colorectal foreign bodies which can be inserted are limited only by the human imagination and have been reported to include bottles, light bulbs, apples, cucumbers, salamis, vibrators, dildos, ice picks, and screwdrivers. Despite the curiosity aroused by these patients, there is a great need to treat them with dignity, keeping in mind the substantial embarrassment they already feel.

3. Depending on the object, various instruments will be required for removal. If there is no evidence of peritonitis, most objects can be removed transanally in the Emergency Department. In order to remove any foreign body of substantial size, anal sphincter relaxation will be necessary. This is accomplished by infiltration of local anesthetics. Utilizing a 25- to 30-gauge needle, a continuous wheal is raised around the anus, usually

requiring around 10 cc of 1% lidocaine or 0.5% bupivicaine. Next, with a finger inserted in the rectum as a guide, a 22-gauge 1½-inch needle is inserted into the anterior and posterior midline as well as left and right midlateral positions, with approximately 2.5 cc of anesthetic injected submucosally in each quadrant. Anal sphincter relaxation should be obtained in about 3 minutes. The local anesthetic can be supplemented with intravenous analgesia and diazepam when necessary.

Following adequate anesthesia, a retractor (e.g., Park's retractor, small gynecologic speculum) is inserted into the rectum. It is best to remove all foreign bodies under direct visualization. Depending on the object, long Kelly hemostats or ring forceps can be utilized to grab the object. It is often useful to insert a 24 F Foley above the object. This can serve two purposes: (1) it helps inhibit further migration of the foreign body and (2) large foreign bodies will often create a vacuum which can be broken by insufflating air into the Foley.

A glass foreign body represents a special problem. Various remedies for removal include utilizing two large kitchen spoons, tonsils snares, or applying a strong adhesive to the object and attaching a "handle" to this. As in removal of all foreign bodies, the emergency physician should set a time limit on retrieval.

Often, just by waiting, the foreign body will descend to the lower part of the rectum where it can be more easily removed. Cathartics and enemas should not be employed. If the object cannot be removed without difficulty, the patient should be admitted, and the surgeon can decide if the object can be removed transanally under general anesthesia or if a laparotomy is required. Any patient with a colorectal foreign body and peritoneal signs requires admission.

If the object is successfully removed in the Emergency Department, careful sigmoidoscopic examination of the rectum is necessary to ensure mucosal integrity.

4. Perforation of the rectum, whether occult or iatrogenic, is the most serious complication of colorectal foreign bodies. Fever, abdominal pain, rectal bleeding, or tenderness should arouse suspicion of perforation. If a sigmoidoscope inspection is inconclusive, flat and upright x-rays of the abdomen as well as chest x-ray should be taken to search for free air. Free air under the diaphragm suggests colonic perforation, while retroperitoneal air suggests rectal perforation. If perforation is still strongly suspected and cannot be visualized on sigmoidoscopic examination and plain x-ray evidence is lacking, a gastrograffin enema should be considered.

Perforation can be divided into two types: (1) perforations above the peritoneal reflection and (2) perforations below the peritoneal reflection. Usually perforations above the peritoneal reflection or intraperitoneal tears will present early with signs and symptoms such as abdominal pain, fever, tachycardia, and peritoneal irritation. Perforations below the peritoneal reflection, extraperitoneal, can be difficult to diagnose. Manifestations of extraperitoneal penetration may not be immediately evident and can range from perirectal abscesses to Fournier's gangrene (fulminating gangrene of the perirectal region).

If rectal perforation is a possibility, the patient should be admitted for observation and started on broad-spectrum antibiotics which cover normal bowel flora. These patients also need tetanus prophylaxis if not current, since clostridium tetanus is found in feces. When abdominal perforation is confirmed or strongly suspected, the patient needs to be taken to the operating room for definitive care.

Other complications of colorectal foreign bodies include mucosal tears and anal sphincter disruption. Small nonbleeding lacerations and abrasions do not require definitive treatment other than local wound care. A tear confined to the subcutaneous tissue that is actively bleeding should be irrigated and coapted with absorbable suture. If the anal sphincter is disrupted, the patient should be taken to the operating room for definitive repair. Otherwise, if perforation and sphincter tears are excluded after removal of a foreign body, the patient should be observed for 4 to 6 hours and discharged with follow-up in 24 hours.

PEARLS:

1. A sentinel skin tag at the posterior or anterior midline usually indicates an underlying rectal fissure.

2. A fissure not located in the midline should arouse suspicion of underlying disease such as inflammatory bowel disease, infection, or cancer.

3. An upright chest x-ray is the most sensitive roentgenogram for intraperitoneal free air.

4. Slight asymmetry of the buttocks can indicate an underlying ischiorectal abscess.

5. Bleeding associated with hemorrhoids in cirrhotics can be very difficult to control.

PITFALLS:

1. Do not discharge patients with rectal pain and fever.

2. Respect the patient's confidentiality. Patients with rectal foreign bodies often become objects of curiosity.

3. Do not use cathartics or enemas in an attempt to remove colorectal foreign bodies.

4. Do not fail to perform a sigmoidoscope examination after removal of a foreign body.

5. Review the differential diagnosis before attributing rectal bleeding to hemorrhoids in patients over 35 years old.

6. Falsely positive guaiac card results can be obtained when iodide, cupric sulfates, ferrous sulfate, ferrous chloride and bromide are present. On the other hand, substances such as vitamin C, activated charcoal, and magnesium-containing antacids can decrease the sensitivity of the guaiac card.

REFERENCES:

Brenner BE, Simon RR. Anorectal emergencies. Ann Emerg Med 1983;12:367-376.

Busch DB, Starling JR. Rectal foreign bodies: case reports and a comprehensive review of the world's literature. Surgery 1986;100(3):512-519.

Crass RA, Tranbaugh RF, Kuds KA, Trunkey DD. Colorectal foreign bodies and perforation. Am J Surg 1981;142:85-88.

Grogel HK. Substances that interfere with guaiac card test: implications for gastric aspirate testing. Am J Emerg Med 1989;7(5):474.

Sonn W, Weinstein MA, Robbin RO. Anorectal disorders. Curr Prob Surg 1983;10(1):1-66.

A NURSE WITH A NEEDLESTICK

Case 31:

A 25-year-old nurse presented to the emergency department at 3:00 am stating that she had sustained a needlestick injury 20 minutes earlier. The needlestick occurred during a cardiopulmonary arrest in the cardiac care unit. The patient did not survive; he was a 46-year-old male who was admitted for chest pain. The hepatitis and HIV status of the patient were unknown. The nurse reluctantly stated that she had not received the hepatitis B vaccination. She also added that she heard the patient was homosexual and was concerned about the possibility of contracting AIDS. The nurse stated she had tested negative for HIV approximately 11 months earlier during an insurance physical. Her last tetanus booster was 3 years ago.

On physical examination, she was an anxious white female in no acute distress. Vital signs revealed a blood pressure of 130/80, a pulse rate of 96/minute and regular, a respiratory rate of 20/minute, and an oral temperature of 98.8° F. Examination of the heart, lungs, and abdomen was unremarkable. Examination of the extremities was notable for a 0.5-cm superficial laceration on the volar aspect of the right index finger.

QUESTIONS:

1. Discuss the general management of puncture wounds.
2. What are the current recommendations regarding hepatitis prophylaxis?
3. What is the risk of HIV transmission? Does HIV prophylaxis exist?

ANSWERS:

1. In many hospitals, the initial evaluation and management of puncture wounds is performed in the Emergency Department. Through proper initial management, it may be possible to prevent subsequent complications and alleviate worries. In evaluating puncture wounds, the physician must address two important points: (1) whether the puncture wound is clean or contaminated and (2) the location. The latter point is important because puncture wounds of the foot have a higher propensity for infection, particularly with Pseudomonas aeruginosa when the puncture occurs through an athletic shoe.

Needlesticks from hospital equipment are usually considered "clean" sticks. Local therapy should include proper irrigation, gentle exploration of the site to determine if there is a retained foreign body (an x-ray should be obtained if there exists any doubt), application of an antiseptic solution, and ascertaining that tetanus immunization is current. The importance of occupational needlestick to health care workers lies in the possibility of transmission of viral disease.

2. The need for postexposure prophylaxis is based on the following factors: (1) whether the source of the blood or body fluid is known, (2) whether the hepatitis B surface antigen status (Hb_sAg) of the source is known, (3) what the hepatitis B vaccination status of the exposed patient is, and (4) whether a vaccinated patient has adequate antibody levels.

Direct percutaneous inoculation by contaminated needle is one of the principle modes of transmission of hepatitis B and non-A, non-B hepatitis. While exact percentages cannot be computed, studies have shown the risk of transmission of hepatitis to be about 1 in 20 (compared to HIV where the rates of transmission is believed to be around 1 in 250) for a single needlestick from a contaminated source.

The following summarizes current recommendations regarding hepatitis B prophylaxis, although there exists controversy over the need to test patients for hepatitis B antibodies before administering the vaccine:

- If the patient is unvaccinated against hepatitis B and the source is known to be positive for hepatitis B, give hepatitis B immunoglobulin (HBIg) 0.06 cc/kg up to 5 cc in the adult in the first 48 hours. Also recommend to the patient that he or she receive the first dose of the hepatitis vaccine within the week. It is well-accepted that the combined use of HBIg and vaccine immediately after exposure to the hepatitis B surface antigen (HB_sAg) carrier provides improved protection against hepatitis B.

- If the source is known and considered to be high risk (e.g., dialysis patient, intravenous drug addict, homosexual) but blood testing is not available within the first 48 hours and the patient is unvaccinated, give HBIg and recommend initiation of the vaccine series.

• If the source is unknown and the donor is considered low risk, HBIg is usually not required. However, this needs to be discussed in detail with the patient. Also, recommend initiation of the vaccine series.

• If the patient is vaccinated, and the donor source is either HB_sAg positive or high risk, check the titer of hepatitis B antibodies. If the titer is greater than 10 SRU by RIA, no further action is warranted. If the titer is inadequate, the physician may proceed as if the patient were unvaccinated. However, this is somewhat controversial as some authorities would recommend just a booster dose of the vaccine.

All patients with possible hepatitis exposure should have follow-up arranged as well as careful documentation of the exposure. Patients exposed to a positive HB_sAg source need either the second vaccine shot in a month or a second dose of HBIg. In addition, some physicians also offer immunoglobulin as a possible protection against non-A, non-B hepatitis. Other possible modes of transmission of hepatitis to the health care worker include indirect percutaneous inoculation of infective plasma or serum, such as through cuts or abrasions or through the mucous membranes.

3. Perhaps no other disease has generated as much controversy as human immunodeficiency virus. One of the most compelling issues is the risk of HIV transmission to health care providers. While the risk of transmission from a single needlestick is considered low (less than 1%), it is the unknown course of the disease and the possibility of transmission of the disease to loved ones that causes much of the anxiety.

If a health care worker has a parenteral or mucous membrane contact with blood or other fluids of a patient, the source should be asked for permission to test his or her blood for HIV. The source patient needs to be made aware of the consequences of testing and offered pretesting counseling. The health care worker will also need to be tested initially to document preexposure HIV status and to be offered pretest counseling. Exact regulations vary in different states as well as different hospitals. It must be kept in mind that it is possible for the source to be HIV positive but still test negative for the antibody early in the course of infection.

If the source patient is proven or known to be HIV positive, or refuses testing, or the contaminated source is unknown, the exposed health care worker should be advised to have bloods drawn initially for HIV testing and repeated at 3 months, 6 months and 1 year. Of the known cases of HIV transmission to health care workers from occupational exposure, all have converted to HIV positive status by 6 months. Many have demonstrated a characteristic viral syndrome around 6 to 12 weeks after exposure.

In addition to the above, once a known significant exposure to possible HIV infected body fluids has occurred, the exposed health care worker should be advised to refrain from any activities which could transmit the virus until his or her status is clarified.

The issue of whether zidovudine (AZT) should be offered as prophylaxis following significant HIV exposure is both controversial and complex. There is currently a lack of definitive information, although clinical trials are under way. It must be kept in mind that the natural history of HIV infection is multifactorial and related to infectious dose, route of infection, and immunocompetence of the individual, thus any intervention will vary among individuals. In general, it would appear that the earlier the initiation of prophylaxis, the more optimal the outcome. However, since AZT is not approved for prophylactic use, the physician must obtain informed consent, with particular attention to information about the short- and long-term side effects of AZT, including blood dyscrasias, headache, myalgias, and fatigue. The current dosage employed is 200 mg every 4 hours for 42 days.

PEARLS:

1. Use gloves, gowns, masks, and eye protection for any patient in whom you may be exposed to body fluids by splash, spray, or heavy bleeding.

2. Health care professionals, renal dialysis patients, institutionalized patients, male homosexuals, sexual partners of HB_sAg positive patients, and neonates of HB_sAg positive mothers should all be immunized against hepatitis.

3. The cost of HBIg ranges from $400 to $600.

4. Immunoglobulin at 0.07 cc/kg (up to 5 cc in the adult) may help prevent the transmission of non-A, non-B hepatitis.

5. Puncture wounds of the foot, particularly through athletic shoes, are predisposed to a higher incidence of Pseudomonas infections.

PITFALLS:

1. Failure to employ universal precautions for all patients can be a serious oversight. Studies have shown that many patients with HIV infection may not be detected or suspected.

2. Never, never recap needles. This is the most common cause of needlesticks.

3. Do not administer the hepatitis vaccine in the buttocks, as this mode of administration has a higher failure rate than if the vaccine is administered in the deltoid.

4. Do not fail to provide follow-up for all patients with possible hepatitis or HIV exposure.

REFERENCES:

Baker JL. What is the occupational risk to emergency care providers from human immunodeficiency virus? Ann Emerg Med 1988;17(7):700-703.

Center for Disease Control. Update: universal precautions for prevention of transmission of HIV, hepatitis B virus, and other blood borne pathogens in health settings. MMWR 1988;37:379-387.

Henderson DK, Gerberdig JL. Prophylactic zidovudine after occupational exposure to human immunodeficiency virus: an internal analysis. J Infect Dis 1989;160(2):321-327.

Kelen GD, Fritz S, Qaguish B, et al. Unrecognized human immunodeficiency in emergency department patients. N Engl J Med 1988;319:1645-1680.

Marcus R: Surveillance of health care workers exposed to blood from patients infected with human immunodeficiency virus. N Engl J Med 1988; 319: 1118-1123.

Trott A: Hepatitis B exposure and the emergency physician. Am J Emerg Med 1987; 5: 54-61.

A VIOLENT YOUNG MAN WITH HYPERTHERMIA

Case 32:

A muscular young male who appeared to be in his mid-twenties was brought to the Emergency Department in handcuffs. According to the accompanying police officers, the patient was found to be "wildly agitated" at an outdoor summer gathering. In the Emergency Department the patient was loud and abusive as he struggled to free himself from the handcuffs. The triage nurse was only able to take the patient's pulse rate which was 120/minute. Quick inspection revealed an agitated, aggressive young male; his skin was diaphoretic, his pupils were approximately 6 mm. The remainder of the physical examination could not be completed because of the patient's extreme agitation.

DIAGNOSTIC CLUES:

Urine dipstick: Strongly positive for occult blood

Urine microscopic examination: No red blood cells noted

Urine toxicology screen: Positive for benzoylecgonine

QUESTIONS:

1. How should the physician proceed in the management of this patient?

2. What is the most likely diagnosis?

3. Discuss the significance and management of an elevated temperature in this patient.

4. What is the implication of a urine that tests strongly positive for occult blood with no red blood cells seen on microscopic examination?

ANSWERS:

1. Nothing can disrupt an Emergency Department more quickly than an agitated, screaming, violent patient. Only preplanned strategies will insure proper management of this patient. The first priority in dealing with a violent patient is to ensure protection of the staff and to protect the patient from himself. A good rule of thumb is that if the patient is not calm enough to obtain accurate vital signs, further measures are necessary to obtain control of the situation. If talking to the patient in a calm and nonthreatening manner is not successful, physical restraints are usually necessary. Never place yourself between the patient and the exit. Ideally, a five member security team should be employed, where one member is assigned to each limb and a team leader to the head. It is best to use leather restraints and place the patient in a prone or lateral decubitus position to help prevent aspiration.

In general, when a patient is extremely agitated, some sort of chemical `restraint' will be necessary in order to adequately assess the patient. For psychotic patients, haloperidol, a butyrophenone, can be utilized. If the patient is known to be in alcohol withdrawal or the history is strongly suggestive of drug toxicity, then benzodiazepines are the drugs of choice. Always use the intravenous route if possible.

Once the patient's agitation is adequately controlled, immediate attention is directed to determine the etiology of the patient's delirium. As in all Emergency Department patients, this initial management includes assessment and stabilization of the airway, breathing, and circulation as well as cervical spine stabilization if there is a question of trauma. All vital signs, including an accurate body temperature, must be obtained and constantly reassessed. Since there is an alteration in the level of consciousness, the patient should be given 50% dextrose in water (D50), naloxone, thiamine, and oxygen. The administration of these four agents is based on the premise that although they may not always help, they will cause no harm. A fingerstick glucose should be performed <u>prior</u> to administration of dextrose.

In addition, blood should be obtained for electrolytes, glucose, BUN, and calcium. Further testing, such as toxicology samples, complete blood count, arterial blood gases, EKG, CAT of the head, and cerebrospinal fluids analysis may all be necessary, depending on the clinical presentation. The major objective at this stage is to separate out organic etiologies such as toxic-metabolic or structural-neurologic disease from functional or psychiatric disorders.

After this patient was appropriately restrained and sedated, the vital signs revealed a pulse rate of 120/minute, blood pressure of 180/110, respiratory rate of 22/minute, and temperature 105.8° F. There was no external evidence of head trauma, the pupils were now 7 mm, equal and reactive to light, and the fundoscopic examination was unremarkable. The patient did have a gag reflex. The neck was supple. The remainder of the physical examination was unremarkable except for some abrasions on the volar aspect of the wrist and forearms. There were no track marks.

Appropriate blood and urine studies were ordered. A lumbar puncture was obtained revealing clear spinal fluid, with a cell count of 2 red blood cells and 0 white blood cells. The protein was 60 mg/dL and the glucose was 70 mg/dL (serum glucose of 96 mg/dL).

2. The patient with a fever and altered mental status presents a true diagnostic challenge. Possible etiologies include infectious disorders such as meningitis, encephalitis, metabolic disorders such as thyrotoxicosis, and thermoregulatory disorders such as heat stroke, head trauma, and drug intoxication. In our patient, the symptomatic signs of agitation, mydriasis, tachycardia, and hypertension along with the presence of benzoylecgonine, the principal metabolite of cocaine, strongly suggests cocaine toxicity. However, this should not preclude the performance of a lumbar puncture.

3. Hyperthermia is the most important prognostic indicator of cocaine mortality, and must be treated aggressively. Cocaine produces an elevated body temperature by several mechanisms, including increased heat production secondary to seizures and agitation, increased calorigenic activity of the liver, and possibly a direct effect on the thermoregulatory center. If a temperature greater than 105° F is recorded, the patient needs to be rapidly cooled. Extreme elevation of temperature will quickly lead to cardiovascular collapse, renal failure, hepatic necrosis, coma, and disseminated intravascular coagulopathy (DIC).

Management should begin with complete control of agitation with benzodiazepines, removal of all clothing, and aggressive cooling via ice water bath immersion or utilization of water sprays and fans. Cooling measures should be stopped at 102° F, but the clinician should continue to monitor the temperature for rebound hyperthermia. Acetaminophen, salicylates, and dantrolene (used in neuroleptic malignant syndrome) are not useful in hyperthermia secondary to cocaine.

4. While cardiac and neurologic complications of cocaine intoxication are well-documented, there has been an increasing awareness of cocaine's effect on various organ systems. The exact pathophysiology of cocaine-induced rhabdomyolysis is not clearly understood, but the resulting complications of acute renal failure and DIC are reported with increasing frequency. Prompt recognition is essential in preventing the ensuing complications of rhabdomyolysis.

Rhabdomyolysis may be suspected by the detection of myoglobin within the urine. The urine will often test positive for blood with benzidine or ortholuidine test strips, but no red blood cells will be seen on the microscopic examination. However, the presence of myoglobin in the urine is often transitory and is affected by a number of factors. Measurement of serum creatinine phosphokinase (CPK) represents the most sensitive method of diagnosing rhabdomyolysis; only when the CPK is normal can rhabdomyolysis be ruled out. The mainstay of treatment is early aggressive volume expansion and forced diuresis with either mannitol and/or furosemide. While advocated by many clinicians, the use of bicarbonate to alkalinize the urine remains controversial.

PEARLS:

1. A useful mnemonic for any patient with an altered mental status is TIPPS on VOWELS.

TIPPS:

T= trauma, tumor, temperature

I= infection

P= psychiatric

P= poison

S= space occupying lesions, stroke, shock, subarachnoid hemorrhage, seizure

VOWELS:

A= alcohol

E= endocrine, exocrine, electrolytes

I= insulin

O= oxygen, opiates

U= uremia (renal disease)

2. While anticholinergic overdoses can produce a similar clinical picture to cocaine/sympathomimetic toxicity (i.e., tachycardia, hyperpyrexia, agitation, dilated pupils), subtle clues such as dry skin and decreased bowel sounds are usually present with anticholinergic overdoses but not seen with sympathomimetic overdoses.

3. Hyperthermia is the single most important correlate of cocaine mortality.

4. A quick test to help differentiate between myoglobin versus hemoglobin in the urine is to look at the spun serum. With myoglobin the serum will be clear, but with hematuria secondary to hemolysis the serum will be pink because of the binding of the hemoglobin with haptoglobin.

PITFALLS:

1. Failure to consider trauma and infection in the presumed overdose patient can be a serious oversight. Fully 25% of all patients who die from supposed overdoses die from infection, with another 25% actually succumbing to traumatic causes.

2. Phenothiazines should not be used routinely to control agitated behavior. They often cause hypotension, potentiate anticholinergic symptoms, and can lower the seizure threshold.

3. Do not induce emesis in a patient with an altered mental status, as they often precipitously lose all airway reflexes or can seize leading to aspiration.

4. Do not fail to reassess the agitated, confused patient. One examination is never enough.

5. Do not forget to write orders for restraints. In many states, this is a requirement.

REFERENCES:

Flomenbaum N, Goldfrank LR, Kulberg AG, Weisman RS. General management of the poisoned or overdosed patient. In: Goldfrank LR, Flomenbaum NE, Lewin NA, et al., eds. Goldfrank's toxicologic emergencies. Norwalk, CT: Appleton-Century-Crofts, 1986:5-28.

Levenson JL. Dealing with the violent patient. Postgrad Med 1985;78(5):329-335.

Roth D, Alarcon FJ, Fernandez JA, et al. Acute rhabdomyolysis associated with cocaine intoxication. N Engl J Med 1988;319:673-677.

Vassallo SV, Delaney KA. Pharmacologic effects on thermoregulation: mechanisms of drug related heat stroke. Clin Toxicol 1989;27:199-224.

Young GP. The agitated patient in the Emergency Department. Emerg Clin North Am 1987;5(11):765-781.

GROIN PAIN IN A YOUNG MALE

Case 33:

A 26-year-old male presented to the triage desk stating that he had been having groin pain for 1 week. He denied any history of trauma, urinary symptoms, or penile discharge. He had no chronic medical problems, had been treated for gonorrhea 2 years earlier, and denied intravenous drug abuse (although he did "smoke" cocaine occasionally).

On examination, the patient was afebrile with stable vital signs. The physical examination was unremarkable, except for inspection of the genitalia which revealed a nonindurated, painful, necrotic ulcer on the shaft of the penis. In addition, there was right inguinal adenopathy, which was tender to palpation. A VDRL was negative.

DIAGNOSTIC CLUE:

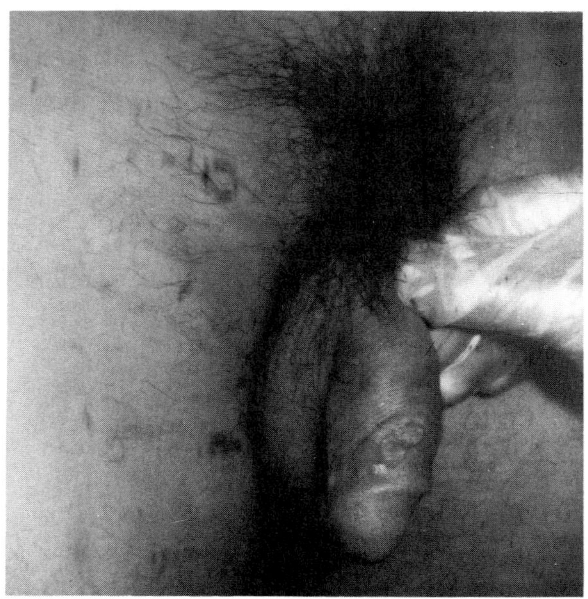

QUESTIONS:

1. What is the tentative diagnosis?
2. What treatment is indicated?
3. Discuss the differential diagnosis.

ANSWERS:

1. The history and physical examination are most consistent with the diagnosis of chancroid. Although it is not well-recognized in the United States, there have been increasing reports in many American cities. In most outbreaks, prostitutes are found to be the reservoir of infection. Worldwide, chancroid is more common than syphilis.

The causative organism is Haemophilus ducreyi, a Gram-negative pleomorphic bacillus. Typically, the patient presents with a painful genital lesion (usually singular in males and three or more lesions in females) that has a necrotic base and nonindurated edges. Lymphadenopathy occurs in about 50% of patients, typically unilateral and ipsilateral to the penile lesion.

While chancroid is not a life-threatening disease, it is of concern because of its established role in the transmission of the human immunodeficiency virus (HIV). Genital ulcerations are thought to provide a means of entry for HIV infection and to facilitate the passage of HIV into vaginal secretions.

2. The drugs of choice to treat chancroid are erythromycin 500 mg orally four times a day for 7 days or ceftriaxone 250 mg IM once. Single dose ceftriaxone may not be adequate in patients with HIV/AIDS. Trimethoprim-sulfamethoxazole 160 mg/800 mg used to be the recommended drug, but there have been increasing reports of resistance.

Once treated, genital ulcers should heal within 7 days and disappear completely within 30 days. Bubos and inguinal adenopathy may take several weeks to resolve. If there is fluctuance to the inguinal adenopathy, the lesion may be aspirated. However, these lesions should NOT be incised and drained because this not only prolongs healing time but may promote fistula formation.

Amoxicillin/clavulanate potassium (Augmentin) and ciprofloxacin have been used effectively outside the United States.

3. Ulcerative lesions of the genitalia are common problems seen in most Emergency Departments. The differential diagnosis should include chancroid, genital herpes, syphilis, granuloma inguinale, lymphogranuloma venereum, and trauma. Most lesions have characteristic traits:

Chancroid	Ulcers are painful, purulent, nonindurated with irregular edges
Syphilis	Associated with painless ulcers that are indurated with a clean base

Herpes	Appears as multiple small grouped vesicles that can coalesce and form shallow painful ulcers--herpes is also associated with painful adenopathy
Lymphogranuloma venereum	While associated with anal strictures, it can also appear as small shallow lesions (which are transient) and prominent inguinal adenopathy (creating a "groove sign")
Granuloma inguinale	A more indolent infection due to <u>Calymmatobacterium (donovaniosis) granulomatis</u>, it is characterized by an extensive, shallow, beefy red ulceration, and the advancing border has a characteristic rolled edge of granulation tissue

Despite these characteristic features, making the diagnosis of ulcerative lesions purely on clinical grounds can be difficult at best. Chancroid is misdiagnosed in up to 30% of the cases. All patients with a genital ulcer should undergo serologic testing for syphilis (VDRL or RPR), cultures for herpes simplex virus, and cultures for <u>H. ducreyi</u>, as well as dark field examination and Gram stain of the ulcer exudate. This will ensure proper diagnosis and treatment.

<u>PEARLS:</u>

1. Solitary painless ulcers on the penis should be considered primary syphilis until proven otherwise.

2. Unilateral adenopathy with chancroid is almost always ipsilateral to the side of the lesion on the shaft of the penis.

3. The presence of chancroid is an established risk factor for the acquisition of human immunodeficiency virus.

<u>PITFALLS:</u>

1. Do not fail to explain to the patient the role of sexual transmission of these diseases.

2. Do not rely on gross appearance of lesions. Many patients have atypical lesions or superinfected ulcerations.

3. Do not incise bubos associated with chancroid. This will prolong healing time and also lead to fistula formation.

4. Dual infections with penile ulcerations are common, such as the presence of both herpes and syphilis, or gonorrhea or chlamydia infection concomitant with penile ulceration.

5. Do not forget to test for syphilis in all cases of sexually transmitted disease since a concurrent infection may well be present.

REFERENCES:

Abramowicz M, ed. Treatment of sexually transmitted diseases. Med Lett 1988;32:5-10.

Chapel TA. How reliable is the morphological diagnosis of penile ulcerations. Sex Transm Dis 1977;(Oct.-Dec.):150-152.

Ronald AR, Plummer F. Chancroid--a newly important sexually transmitted disease. Arch Dermatol 1989;125:1413-1418.

Salzman RS, Kraus SJ, Klans RG. Chancroid ulcers that are not chancroid: causes and epidemiology. Arch Dematol 1984;120:636-639.

Schmid GP, Sanders LL, Blount JH, Alexander RE. Chancroid in the United States: reestablishment of an old disease. JAMA 1987;258:3265-3268.

TRAUMA IN PREGNANCY

Case 34:

A 21-year-old G2P1001 female presented to the Emergency Department 12 weeks pregnant complaining of abdominal pain. She had been kicked in the epigastrium and right chest by a mugger approximately 2 hours prior to presentation. The patient denied shortness of breath, nausea, or vaginal bleeding. Past medical history included a recent uncomplicated urinary tract infection treated successfully with oral antibiotics and cesarean section at age 19.

Physical examination revealed a thin female in no distress. The blood pressure was 110/70, the heart rate was 86/minute and the respiratory rate was 24/minute. The chest was clear to auscultation. There was a 4-cm ecchymotic area over the right lower breast. The abdomen was mildly tender in the epigastrium and right lower quadrant. There was no blood in the vaginal vault. The cervix was tender to lateral motion and the os was closed. The uterus was 12 to 14 weeks in size and slightly tender; the adnexa were normal. The rectal examination, including guaiac test, was normal. Laboratory studies including complete blood count, electrolyte profile, hepatic enzymes, and serum amylase were within normal limits. An open-technique supraumbilical peritoneal lavage revealed 10 cc of gross blood.

DIAGNOSTIC CLUES:

1. Fetal heart tones were noted to be absent.

2. Ultrasound revealed an irregularity at the fundus of the uterus.

QUESTIONS:

1. What is the diagnosis?

2. What is the most common mechanism of injury leading to this condition?

3. What is the value of the history and physical examination in the pregnant trauma victim?

4. What diagnostic tests are useful in trauma in pregnancy?

5. Outline the management of the pregnant trauma patient.

ANSWERS:

1. The diagnosis is uterine rupture.

2. Traumatic rupture of the uterus is a relatively uncommon event and generally requires tremendous forces such as a motor vehicle accident. Motor vehicle accidents account for 50 to 85% of blunt trauma incurred during pregnancy. Traumatic uterine rupture usually occurs when the victim is ejected from the vehicle, with a rapid deceleration over the seat belt, or when the seat belt is placed improperly over the fundus.

The effects of automobile restraint systems have been evaluated. It has been hypothesized that a lap belt focuses the force of deceleration on the pelvis and, with forward flexion of the mother's body, compresses the uterus between the spine and the belt. A sudden increase in pressure may cause the uterus to rupture. Previous uterine surgery increases the risk of uterine rupture. Since scars are avascular, these patients present less dramatically than do patients without prior surgery. Therefore, lap belts theoretically increase fetal morbidity.

However, lap belts have been shown to protect the mother from injury and actually decrease maternal and fetal morbidity. The addition of the shoulder harness has increased fetal survival from 50 to 92% compared to the standard lap belt restraint.

The anatomic and physiologic changes which accompany pregnancy increase the likelihood of catastrophic trauma. The pregnant abdomen makes a larger target for assault leading to blunt and penetrating injuries. The gravid uterus is at risk for rupture, contusion, or laceration. The blood supply to the uterus and bladder is markedly increased and injury may lead to extensive intra- or retroperitoneal hemorrhage.

3. The inaccuracy of the initial clinical impression in patients suspected of having blunt abdominal injuries has been reported to range from 16 to 45%. Abdominal symptoms and signs are often diminished, delayed, or absent in pregnant women with blunt abdominal injuries. Often patients will complain only of mild abdominal pain. Vaginal bleeding suggests placental abruption or uterine rupture, but approximately 20% of these cases have no external bleeding.

Hemodynamic changes during pregnancy make vital signs and cardiopulmonary status difficult to interpret. At approximately 10 weeks gestation, there is a rise in red blood cell mass and an even greater rise in plasma volume, leading to a dilutional anemia. By the third trimester, the maternal blood volume is expanded by 45% and is maintained at that level for the remainder of the pregnancy. The maternal cardiac output is increased by 1.0 to 1.4 L/minute during the first 10 weeks of gestation. While there is a rise in blood volume, there is a marked increase in peripheral blood flow secondary to vasodilation.

Therefore, a pregnant woman will have a lower blood pressure, lower central venous pressure, and warm skin. The pregnant woman can tolerate a 30 to 35% loss of blood volume without changing her mean arterial pressure because of the high plasma volume. However, this blood loss leads to 10 to 20% reduction in uterine blood flow. Therefore, a normotensive patient may give the physician a false sense of security when in fact the fetus is in distress. Because of peripheral vasodilation, the cold and clammy skin of shock may not be present in the pregnant woman.

The heart rate increases throughout pregnancy so that a normal pulse rate is 80 to 90 beats/minute even at rest. The respiratory rate can be deceptive since minute ventilation is increased by 50% during pregnancy. The pCO_2 should be approximately 30 mm Hg and normocapnia indicates significant hypoventilation. A lower functional residual capacity and higher oxygen consumption during pregnancy predisposes the mother to hypoxemia with a brief interruption of respiratory function. Hypoxemia decreases placental blood flow by stimulating catecholamine release that leads to vasoconstriction. Therefore, the effects of maternal hypoxemia are magnified in the fetus.

Physical examination of the abdomen is less sensitive in pregnancy. There is compartmentalization of the abdominal organs as they are displaced by the gravid uterus. Rebound tenderness and guarding as signs of intraabdominal injury may be diminished as the peritoneum and abdominal musculature are stretched by the enlarging uterus. The uterus and bladder are displaced and become abdominal organs. By the 12th week of gestation, they are no longer protected by the bony pelvis and are more prone to injury.

A pelvic exam may reveal uterine size-date discrepancy, uterine tenderness or bleeding, or leakage of amniotic fluid. However, even significant uterine, placental, or fetal injury may have unimpressive physical findings.

Doppler measurements of fetal cardiac activity and monitoring of uterine activity can often detect significant injuries in the pregnant woman who appears clinically normal. Four hours of continuous cardiotocographic monitoring after trauma can predict which patients can be expected to have adverse reactions.

4. The decision regarding specific diagnostic testing should be based on anticipated areas of injury. The likelihood that a given organ will be injured in blunt abdominal trauma in the pregnant patient depends on gestational age and mechanism of injury. In early pregnancy, injuries are similar to those in nonpregnant patient. In late pregnancy, uterine rupture and placental abruption are more common.

Simple diagnostic maneuvers provide clues to the nature and extent of injury. Passing of a nasogastric tube for decompression of the stomach will aid respiration and allow examination of the stomach contents. Urinary bladder catheterization obtains urine for examination and for monitoring of urinary output. Simple laboratory studies should include complete blood count, amylase, and liver enzymes.

Plain films should be well-coordinated, as they contribute to radiation risk in pregnancy. However, studies should not be withheld since most diagnostic radiographs have one-tenth the radiation dose limit during pregnancy. Ultrasonography can be used acutely to detect injuries to the liver and spleen as well as to identify blood or fluid adjacent to these organs or in the pelvis. It has not gained favor for initial evaluation because it has a limited repertoire. In the stable patient, laparoscopy alone or with peritoneal lavage might help to specify the location and degree of injury. However, the procedure requires experienced personnel and usually necessitates general anesthesia.

Pregnancy has often been considered a relative contraindication to diagnostic peritoneal lavage. However, in a review of pregnant women who underwent peritoneal lavage by the open midline infra- or supraumbilical approach, the technique was found to be safe and accurate. In the general population, diagnostic peritoneal lavage has been shown to be 98.5% accurate.

Contrast studies have been used to identify specific sites of injury. Computer tomography is most effectively used for the diagnosis of retroperitoneal or pelvic injury. Angiography can determine sites of hemorrhage. Contrast studies of the gastrointestinal tract, urethra, and bladder have identified injuries in these organs.

The transplacental hemorrhage of fetal blood into the maternal circulation has been termed fetomaternal hemorrhage. The incidence of fetomaternal hemorrhage is four to five times higher in injured pregnant women than in uninjured women. Fetomaternal hemorrhage can cause Rh sensitization in the mother and cardiac dysrhythmias, anemia, and death in the fetus.

The Betke-Kleinhauer acid-elution test can detect and quantify fetomaternal hemorrhage. However, the correlation between fetomaternal hemorrhage and the severity of maternal injury is unclear. While the Betke-Kleinhauer test is useful to determine the need for and amount of Rh (D) immunoglobulin to be given the Rh negative woman, its usefulness in the emergency setting has not been studied.

Trauma can cause fetal and maternal compromise in the face of normal diagnostic studies. It has been suggested that, in view of the inaccuracy of the initial clinical impression and unreliability or risk of available diagnostic tests, the traumatized patient should be monitored and observed for at least 4 hours even after minor injuries. External monitor tracings showing changes in or absence of fetal heart rate may be the earliest signs of fetal and maternal compromise. This technique appears to be superior to ultrasonography in the diagnosis of placental abruption and to evaluate fetal well-being.

5. The initial management requires airway maintenance, oxygenation, and controlled ventilation if necessary. Circulation should be maintained with volume replacement and the maintenance of venous return by displacing the gravid uterus from the inferior vena cava. After the 20th week of gestation, the volume of crystalloids should be increased by 50% because of the increase in plasma volume. Blood transfusion should be initiated if stabilization is inadequate with crystalloids. Rh negative blood must be used if Rh antigen status in unknown.

Patients should be placed in the left lateral decubitus position to relieve the pressure of the gravid uterus on the cardiac output. The pneumatic antishock garment (PASG) can improve blood pressure by increasing preload and systemic vascular resistance (afterload), controlling pelvic and abdominal hemorrhage, and mobilizing blood to the upper body. However, inflation of the abdominal compartment can compress the uterus against the inferior vena cava and decrease preload.

After maternal stabilization, the fetal heart rate should be determined and cardiotocograhic monitoring should be instituted. Fetal bradycardia or tachycardia, persistent decelerations, the absence of variability between beats, or the presence of uterine contraindications require emergency obstetric evaluation.

If the mother is Rh negative, Rh (D) immunoglobulin should be administered within 72 hours of the antigenic stimulus.

In the event of cardiac arrest unresponsive to a few minutes of advanced cardiac life support, thoracotomy and open-chest massage should be considered and emergency Caesarean section if the fetus is still viable and over 24 weeks of age. Open-chest massage has been shown to improve cardiac output and to optimize perfusion. Cesarean delivery can improve maternal venous return and can aid in maternal resuscitation.

PEARLS:

1. The recommended ABC's of trauma care given to the nonpregnant trauma patient apply to the trauma patient.

2. Prevention of fetal anoxia is essential to prenatal survival. This is best accomplished by optimizing the mother's respiratory status.

3. Be aware of the normal physiologic changes during pregnancy. Pregnancy is a high-output, low-resistance state in which cardiac output increases up to 40%, heart rate rises 10 to 15 beats per minute, and blood volume increases 30 to 50%. At the same time, there is a drop of 5 to 15 mm Hg in systolic and diastolic pressure in the second trimester.

4. Tetanus prophylaxis (with either toxoid or human tetanus immunoglobulin) is safe during pregnancy and should be administered when indicated.

5. Proper positioning of seat belt during pregnancy can help prevent anterior abdominal wall trauma. The seat belt should be worn encircling the pelvis below the protuberant abdomen, rather than high on the abdomen. Also, the shoulder harness component will decrease the risk of fetal harm.

PITFALLS:

1. Do not fail to recognize the abnormal physiologic changes of pregnancy. Owing to increased blood volume, the pregnant patient in the third trimester may lose 30 to 35% of her blood volume before symptoms of hypotension develop. Heart rate, blood pressure, and pO_2 are unreliable indicators of adequate maternal resuscitation. Serial HCO_3 levels and lactate levels may be more sensitive indicators of adequate perfusion.

2. Remember to position the patient properly. In advanced pregnancy, if the mother is placed in the supine position, the gravid uterus will compress the inferior vena cava, decreasing the preload, and causing hypotension. This can be avoided by placing the patient in the left lateral decubitus position or placing a wedge under the right flank.

3. Do not withhold necessary studies just because the patient is pregnant. Teratogenic levels are rarely reached with routine diagnostic studies (the fetus is most vulnerable between the 9th and 12th week).

4. Do not inflate the abdominal compartment if a PASG is utilized.

5. While a tender hypertonic uterus suggests placental separation, absence of these findings does not exclude the diagnosis.

6. Do not forget to check the Rh status of the mother and administer Rhogam if indicated.

REFERENCES:

Crosby WM, Costiloe JP. Safety of lap-belt restraint for pregnant victims of automobile collisions. N England J Med 1971;284:632-636.

Enden RD, Parker RT, Gall SA. Rupture of the pregnant uterus: a 53 year review. Obst & Gynecol 1986;68:671-674.

Espositos TJ, Gens DR, Gerber-Smith L, Scorpio R. Evaluation of blunt abdominal trauma during pregnancy. J Trauma 1989;29:1628-1632.

Kantz VL, Dotters DJ, Droegemuller W. Perimortem cesarean delivery. Obstet & Gynecol 1986;571-576.

Pearlman MD, Tintinalli JE, Lorenz RP. A prospective controlled study of the outcome after trauma during pregnancy. Am J Obstet Gynecol 1990;162:1502-1510.

SYNCOPE IN A YOUNG FEMALE

Case 35:

A 21-year-old female was brought to the Emergency Department by a friend after she "passed out" at the end of an aerobics class. She stated she noticed some palpitations and felt dizzy before losing consciousness. A witness stated the patient was unconscious for approximately 3 minutes. No seizure activity was noted at the scene. The patient stated this had never happened to her before, and she had been in good health her entire life. Her only medication was birth control pills. Otherwise her medical history was unremarkable except for being told she had a heart murmur when she was a child, and that her father died suddenly from a "heart attack" at age 39. The patient denied any chest pain and stated she became mildly short of breath with exercise.

On physical examination, the patient appeared healthy and in no apparent distress. Vital signs were pulse 60/minute and regular, blood pressure 106/68 without orthostatic changes, and respiratory rate 18/minute and nonlabored. Her chest was clear. Cardiac examination revealed a normal apical impulse, and a grade II/VI systolic ejection along the left sternal border. The murmur increased in intensity with the Valsalva maneuver. The remainder of the examination was unremarkable.

DIAGNOSTIC CLUE:

I aVR V_1 V_4

II aVL V_2 V_5

III aVF V_3 V_6

QUESTIONS:

1. What historical information and findings on physical examination are most important in the evaluation of a patient with syncope?

2. What is the most likely diagnosis of syncope?

3. What is the most likely diagnosis in this patient?

4. Which ancillary tests are most useful in the emergency department in the evaluation of the patient with syncope?

5. Does this patient need to be admitted?

ANSWERS:

1. Syncope is a common presenting complaint in the Emergency Department, accounting on the average for 3% of visits. In most cases syncope is a benign, self-limited event, but it can also be a harbinger of sudden death. It is the duty of the emergency physician to first ensure that a life-threatening illness is not present. Once stabilization of the vital signs (ABC's) is ensured, data gathering can occur.

The first step is to determine if syncope actually occurred. The physician must establish that there was a sudden loss of consciousness with complete recovery. Patients who think they were unconscious for 1 to 2 seconds probably were not. Often much of the history needs to be acquired from bystanders, family, and prehospital personnel.

The history should focus on three essential elements: (1) the presyncopal period, (2) the syncopal period, and (3) the postsyncopal period. The presyncopal period is probably the most important area to focus on. Inquire what the patient was doing before syncope occurred and the position the patient was in. The patient in this case had just finished exercising and was standing before passing out.

Also, ask about premonitory symptoms and their duration. While nausea and sweating are nonspecific, antecedent chest pain or palpitations imply cardiac disease, while vertigo, diplopia, dysarthria, hemiparesis, or aura shift the focus to the nervous system. Little or no warning suggests an arrhythmia or seizure as the etiology. Syncope during recumbency is worrisome and is highly suggestive of a cardiac or neurologic problem.

If the syncopal episode was witnessed, try to obtain information about the patient's condition during and after loss of consciousness. Duration of unconsciousness, color, pulse, respirations, and any seizure activity should be recorded. Cyanosis and respiratory distress during syncope may underlie a cardiopulmonary event, but pallor and clamminess can occur with any type of syncope. If seizure activity was witnessed, determine whether it consisted of repetitive tonic-clonic movements (representing a true seizure) or brief clonic jerking, which is nonspecific. Questions during the postsyncopal period center on fecal or urinary incontinence, postictal confusion, and presence of focal neurologic signs.

Other historical information which helps to differentiate the various etiologies of syncope are a history of being an "easy" fainter, presence of any associated medical illness, current medications, use of alcohol or illicit drugs, family history (particularly familial history of syncope and sudden death), history of a heart murmur, and menstrual history.

The extent and focus of the physical examination is directed by the history. Vital signs should always include orthostatic measurements in the stable patient. Heart rate and blood pressure should be recorded in both supine and standing positions whenever possible. A reflex tachycardia with volume depletion may be blunted by concomitant use of beta blockers. Note the general appearance of the patient, paying particular attention to level of alertness, skin color, and any evidence of trauma. During the cardiopulmonary examination, emphasis is on the presence of murmurs and the effect of the Valsalva maneuver on their intensity, and timing of the carotid upstroke. Any suggestion of syncope secondary to orthostatic hypotension mandates the stool be analyzed for occult blood. A careful neurologic examination is warranted.

The history and physical examination are sufficient to make the diagnosis approximately 50% of the time when an etiology can be determined.

2. After completing the history and physical examination, the physician must formulate a preliminary diagnosis. It is this preliminary diagnosis that will guide future actions such as stabilizing efforts and selection of diagnostic studies. The goal of the Emergency Department evaluation is to differentiate life-threatening causes of syncope from benign etiologies.

Abnormalities of circulatory control are represented by vasovagal or vasodepressor reflex, orthostatic hypotension and carotid hypersensitivity. By far the most common cause of syncope, particularly for patients less than 40 years old, is vasovagal syncope ("fainting"). Usually there will be a precipitating factor (e.g., fear, stress, hunger, pain) leading to vagal stimulation without the normal accompanying sympathetic response. This leads to bradycardia (heart rate 40 to 60 beats/minute) and hypotension (systolic blood pressure 40 to 60 mm Hg) with prodromal symptoms of nausea, queasiness, and lightheadedness. Invariably, the patient was in a standing position before falling; therefore, the emergency care provider needs to be alert for injuries secondary to a fall. Unconsciousness is usually brief, lasting seconds to minutes.

The diagnosis of orthostatic hypotension can be made if a patient's symptoms are reproduced when the patient assumes an upright position and pulse rate increases by 10 or more beats/minute and/or systolic or diastolic pressure falls 20 mm Hg or more. There are many reasons for orthostatic hypotension (e.g., volume depletion secondary to hemorrhage, gastrointestinal fluid loses or overdiuresis, impairment of autonomic nervous system, medications), with the most common being a failure of normal physiologic mechanisms to compensate for venous pooling in the legs when the patient stands upright.

Treatment depends upon the etiology (e.g., replacing fluid losses, discontinuing medications). Sometimes the underlying state causing orthostatic hypotension is irreversible (e.g., autonomic neuropathy due to diabetes) and no definitive therapy exists.

Carotid hypersensitivity represents an exaggerated cardioinhibitory response to carotid stimulation. The diagnosis should be considered in patients who report symptoms of light-headedness and syncope in specific situations such as shaving or backing a car out of the driveway. However, it is important not to jump to conclusions when carotid sinus massage causes periods of asystole, since this can occur in the asymptomatic patient.

Cardiac syncope occurs when the cardiac output is reduced to the point of impairing cerebral perfusion. Most cases of cardiac syncope are apparent or can be strongly suspected on the basis of the history and physical examination. Cardiac syncope is more likely in elderly patients, patients with a cardiac history, and in patients with syncope which occurs abruptly or after physical exertion.

Both tachyarrhythmias and bradyarrhythmias lead to a decreased cardiac output by shortening diastolic filling time, inciting asynchronous atrial contraction (loss of "atrial kick"), and with conditions such as ventricular tachycardia, precipitating asynchronous ventricular contraction. Abrupt reductions in heart rate (e.g., Stokes-Adams heart block) are more likely to manifest as syncope than gradual reductions in heart rate. Cardiac outflow obstructions such as aortic stenosis and hypertrophic cardiomyopathy are associated with effort-related syncope. Pulmonary embolus and myxomas also are examples of cardiac outflow obstruction leading to syncope.

The most common metabolic cause of syncope is hypoglycemia. Hypoxia, hyponatremia, and drug or alcohol intoxication are metabolic derangements which can lead to a transient loss of consciousness. Metabolic abnormalities leading to syncope share the features of gradual onset and resolution of symptoms.

The role of neurologic events in the evolution of syncope is unclear. While generalized seizures clearly cause a transient loss of consciousness, syncope is not a common feature of transient ischemic attack (TIA). When vascular syncope does occur it is usually due to compromise of the vertebrobasilar circulation rather than the anterior carotid arteries. However, with posterior circulation insufficiency, loss of consciousness should not be the sole symptom; there should be other neurologic symptoms such as diplopia, vertigo, dysarthria, and hemiparesis. Diffuse cerebrovascular spasm as is seen with encephalopathy can also lead to a temporary state of unconsciousness.

3. Based on the history and physical examination and corroborated by the EKG, idiopathic hypertrophic subaortic stenosis (IHSS), also known as asymmetric septal hypertrophy (ASH) was suspected. An echocardiogram was obtained in the Emergency Department which showed thickening of the septum in relation to the posterior left ventricle wall and abnormal anterior motion of the mitral leaflet during systole.

IHSS goes by many names--no less than 46 terms! The clinical spectrum is broad and ranges from an incidental asymptomatic findings to sudden death. Symptoms occur when beta adrenergic stimulation such as exercise leads to a dynamic left ventricular outflow obstruction, producing dyspnea, chest pain, syncope, and possibly sudden death. The key physical finding in patients with IHSS is a systolic ejection murmur that increases in intensity when there is a decrease in left ventricular cavity size (e.g., Valsalva, standing, inhalation of amyl nitrates) while the murmur decreases in intensity when there is an increase in left ventricular cavity size (squatting, passive elevation of legs). Recently, concomitant cardiac arrhythmias have been increasingly implicated, particularly in regard to syncope and sudden death. Patients with IHSS do not tolerate supraventricular tachycardia well.

4. A routine battery of tests for all patients who experience a syncopal episode does not exist. The customary use of multiple screening tests and procedures can be both misleading and expensive. Excluding arrhythmias as the cause of the patient's syncopal episode is the biggest challenge. A standard 12-lead EKG and cardiac monitoring are the most accessible and useful early studies. Depending on the findings of the history and physical examination, blood glucose determination, electrolyte studies, and an arterial blood gas may be indicated. If there is any suggestion of volume depletion or if stools are positive for blood, a hematocrit should be obtained.

Further studies are indicated in patients who are strongly suspected to have a cardiac or neurologic origin to their syncope which is not apparent on routine testing. This can include ambulatory EKG monitoring (Holter monitor, electrophysiologic testing), echocardiography, CAT scanning, and electrocardiography.

The important point in testing for syncope is that while diagnostic studies can be most useful, they have a higher predictive value if ordered by a careful history and physical examination.

5. At the conclusion of the history, physical examination and Emergency Department adjunctive studies, the emergency physician must decide the disposition of the patient. Syncopal patients can be placed into one of three categories: (1) low risk, (2) equivocal risk, and (3) high risk. Patients who are at low risk and whose history and physical examination strongly suggest a vasovagal episode can be discharged with follow-up arrangements.

The second group of patients, those whose history or physical examination possibly disclose findings that could account for syncope, pose a more difficult challenge. If there is any question of serious disease or if the patient is elderly, always err on the side of the best interest of the patient. All decisions should be discussed with not only the patient but also the patient's family and private physician. High-risk patients, those with a history and physical examination strongly suggestive of cardiac syncope, should be hospitalized and admitted for cardiac monitoring.

In the patient in question, although admission may not alter future mortality, it will provide the physician and patient the opportunity to explore diagnostic and therapeutic options.

On the other hand, patients who have a documented cardiac etiology to their syncope and experience recurrent syncopal episodes may not benefit from repeat admissions. Again, all decisions must be made with the patient, family, and private physician understanding the nature of the disease and inherent risks.

PEARLS:

1. Patients determined to have a cardiac basis for their syncope have up to a 25% one-year mortality rate.

2. Up to 20% of patients with an acute myocardial infarction may relate a syncopal episode. This may be secondary to a ventricular dysrhythmia or uncompensated drop in cardiac output.

3. If there is a prolonged prodromal period before syncope, think of the six H's: hypoxia, hypoglycemia, hypothyroidism, hypotension, hysteria, and hyperventilation.

4. With an otherwise normal myocardium, syncope resulting from a supraventricular tachycardia is seen in four circumstances: (1) atrial fibrillation, (2) atrial fibrillation in Wolf-Parkinson-White syndrome, (3) atrial flutter with a 1:1 ventricular response, and (4) any supraventricular rhythm with a prolonged sinus node recovery.

5. Patients who state they were unconscious for 1 to 2 secs probably were not!

PITFALLS:

1. Orthostatic changes in blood pressure can take up to five minutes to occur. Don't just measure blood pressure the moment the patient assumes an upright position.

2. Do not forget to inquire why an elderly patient fell.

3. Do not order ancillary test blindly. Let the history and physical examination dictate which studies are necessary.

4. Syncope is not a common feature of TIAs. When the cerebrovascular circulation is the etiological basis, syncope is almost always due to vertebrobasilar ischemia.

REFERENCES:

Day SC, Cook EF, Funkenstein J, Goldman L. Evaluation and outcome of emergency room patients with transient loss of consciousness. Am J Med 1982;73:15-23.

Kapoor WN, Peterson J, Wieand WS, Karpf M. Diagnostic and prognostic implications in patients with syncope. Am J Med 1987;83:700-708.

Linzer M. Syncope. South Med J 1987;80(J):545-553.

Maron BJ, Bonow RO, Cannon RO, et al. Hypertrophic cardiomyopathy--interrelations of clinical manifestations, pathophysiology, and therapy. N Engl J Med 1987;316:780-789.

Martin GJ, Adams SL, Martin HG, et al. Prospective evaluation of syncope in patients presenting to the Emergency Department. Ann Emerg Med 1984;13:499-504.

A PATIENT REFUSING TREATMENT

Case 36:

A male who appeared to be in his late twenties was brought into the Emergency Department by local police officers to have a scalp laceration repaired. According to the police report, the patient was involved in an altercation in a bar where he was a frequent patron.

The patient was initially agitated, belligerent and uncooperative and refused to be examined. As the nurse tried to convince the patient to allow her to take his vital signs, he became unresponsive. After ensuring that the patient evidenced good air exchange and a stable pulse and blood pressure, the physician administered 25 g D50 IV, naloxone 0.8 mg IV, and thiamine 100 mg IV. Approximately 3 minutes later, the patient once again became combative and stated emphatically that he wanted to leave the Emergency Department.

The patient was physically restrained. His vital signs at this point revealed a pulse of 96/minute and regular and blood pressure of 140/92. After vital signs were obtained, the patient again became unresponsive. The naloxone was repeated with no response. The patient did not respond to verbal stimuli and withdrew his left arm and leg to painful stimuli, but did not respond to the same stimulation on the right side. Pupillary examination revealed a right pupil of 6 mm that did not respond to direct or consensual light reflexes; the left pupil was 3 mm and reactive to direct light stimulus. In addition, a 4-cm scalp laceration was noted just anterior to the right ear.

DIAGNOSTIC CLUE:

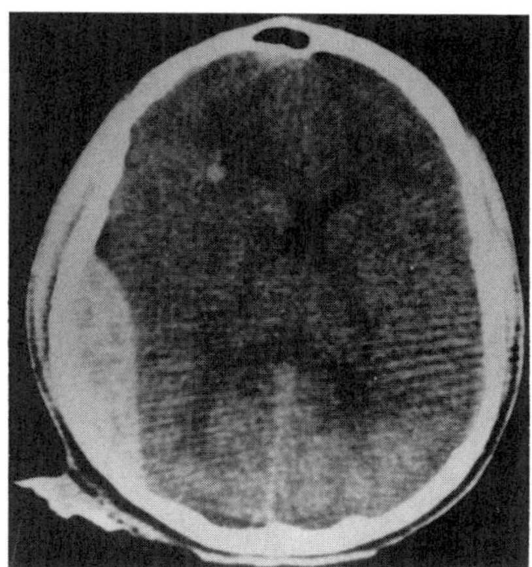

QUESTIONS:

1. What is the diagnosis and how does this account for the patient's neurological status?

2. Did this patient have the right initially to refuse examination and treatment?

3. What signs and symptoms are vital in distinguishing the patient with a severe head injury from one with mild or moderate injury?

4. Discuss airway management in the patient with acute head injury.

5. What diagnostic and therapeutic options are applicable in the ED management of acute head trauma?

ANSWERS:

1. Head trauma serious enough to alter a patient's level of consciousness is due to diffuse axonal injury or a focal lesion (e.g., epidural hematoma, subdural hematoma, intracerebral hemorrhage). The diagnosis is epidural hematoma based on the characteristic appearance on CAT scan of a peripherally located biconvex mass of blood density.

In order to obtain an optimal outcome from head trauma, a basic knowledge of the pathophysiology involved with head injuries is necessary. The skull serves as a rigid container encasing the brain, blood, and cerebrospinal fluid. The tentorium divides the brain into a supratentorial compartment and an infratentorial compartment. A large aperture, the incisura, serves as an exit for the midbrain to pass from the cerebrum.

Any increase in the volume of one compartment of the cranium takes place at the expense of the others, usually being the brain tissue that is displaced. Additionally, with an increase of volume and displacement of brain tissue there is an increase in the intracranial pressure (ICP). This is important because cerebral perfusion pressure (CPP) is determined by the difference between the mean arterial pressure (MAP) and the intracranial pressure (CPP=MAP-ICP). This process is normally "auto-regulated," but trauma to the brain results in a loss of this mechanism.

An epidural hematoma is usually secondary to a laceration of the middle meningeal artery, with bleeding into the space that exists between the inner table of the skull and its periosteum (dura). As the hematoma expands, a predictable sequence of events occurs. The epidural hematoma in this case is located in the temporal lobe region, forcing the uncus (the most medial portion of the temporal lobe) toward the tentorial notch. The third cranial nerve, lying beneath the uncus, is compromised, producing an ipsilateral fixed dilated pupil. In almost all instances, the side with the dilated pupil will indicate the correct side of pathology.

The pupillary changes are almost always preceded by a depression in the level of consciousness, resulting from compression of the small arteries supplying the reticular formation of the brain stem. Further displacement of the uncus causes compression of the pyramidal tracts. Traditionally, this is noted to cause a contralateral hemiparesis or hemiplegia, but in up to one-quarter of the cases the contralateral pyramidal tracts are affected, resulting in ipsilateral weakness. The latter situation is known as a false localizing sign.

Brain herniation may also occur under the falx (cingulate herniation) or through the foramen at the base of the skull (central herniation). The typical scenario seen with an epidural hematoma is an initial period of loss of consciousness resulting from the concussive force, a subsequent "lucid period," and finally the deterioration of mental state seen with uncal herniation.

2. One of the basic premises of our society is that each patient has the right to decide whether he or she wants medical therapy. The responsibility of the physician is to ensure that the patient has a complete understanding of the need for care and possible consequences from delivery or lack of delivery of treatment. This issue is referred to as consent and can be paraphrased as "what the patient wants done at this moment." Consent does not need to be expressed verbally or even in writing. The voluntary presence of a patient in the ED can be considered a form of consent.

However, there are exceptions to the consent rule. Patients intoxicated with alcohol and patients with head trauma fall into the category of implied consent. These are emergency situations where the patient is not considered competent to make a decision. One of the biggest pitfalls in emergency medicine practice is incorrectly attributing the patient's mental status to the effect of alcohol or drugs. When faced with this situation, be guided by the principle of doing what is best for the patient. Careful documentation will protect the physician more than any blood alcohol level. One would do well to heed the words of Sir William Osler, "Better to admit a patient dead drunk than have him return dead sober."

3. Injuries to the head present with a variable and changing clinical picture. Unless a systematic approach is utilized, the clinician can lose sight of the larger picture. The first priority is ensuring stability of the respiratory and cardiovascular systems, the proverbial ABC's. A word of caution--textbooks often speak of associated respiratory patterns with different degrees of head trauma. In actuality this is rarely useful, as the head injured patient often has associated problems such as intoxicants, chest trauma, and shock, which will also influence respiratory parameters.

The initial neurologic examination needs to be both rapid and pertinent. The goal should be to determine the severity of head injury, to determine the baseline neurologic status and to look for signs of focal lesions and/or herniation. Level of consciousness is the most important clinical observation. A good basic screening examination is the AVPU system: the patient is <u>A</u>lert, only responds to <u>V</u>erbal stimulation, only responds to <u>P</u>ainful stimulation, or is <u>U</u>nresponsive. A patient with a <u>mild</u> head injury has no depression in the level of consciousness and lack of neurologic deficit. A <u>moderate</u> head injury implies a depressed level of consciousness but ability to obey at least one verbal command, while a patient with a <u>severe</u> head injury is unable to obey any verbal command.

Perhaps the biggest mistake made in assessing the head-injured patient is reliance on a single neurologic examination. The results of a single examination represent only a point on a curve. More important, the clinician needs to know if the patient is improving or deteriorating. When describing a patient's level of consciousness, try to avoid terms such as obtunded, semicomatose, or lethargic.

The neurologic examination should provide the answer to five questions:

1. Does the patient open his or her eyes and to what stimuli?
2. Does the patient follow commands?
3. Is the patient moving all extremities equally?
4. What is the response to painful stimuli?
5. What is the pupil size and how do the pupils react to bright light?

When evaluating pupil size, be sure to correlate size with the patient's level of consciousness. While a fixed dilated pupil with a decreasing level of consciousness is impending herniation until proven otherwise, the same pupil in a wide awake patient is more likely to be due to local eye trauma or medications.

A useful head trauma assessment scale with prognostic significance is the Glasgow Coma Scale (GCS). The scale is based on three parameters: eye response, motor response, and verbal response. It has been found to have high interobserver reproducibility and requires no equipment.

The GCS score can range from 3 to 15. A GCS of 8 or less is considered a severe head injury, between 9 and 12 a moderate injury, and 13 to 15 is a mild injury. More important are changes in scores. For example, a patient whose GCS drops from 8 to 6 will see a decrease in favorable outcome from a 50% chance to less than 5%. A drawback to the GCS is that it cannot take into account the effect of intoxication with alcohol and drugs, postictal states, or the effects of hypoxia or hypotension and therefore these patients tend to score lower.

GLASGOW COMA SCALE (GCS)

Parameter	Stimulus	Score
Eye		
	Opens spontaneously	4
	Opens to voice	3
	Opens to pain	2
	No response	1
Motor		
	Obeys commands	6
	Localizes painful stimulus	5
	Withdraws from painful stimulus	4
	Decorticate posturing in response to pain	3
	Decerebrate posturing in response to pain	2
	No response to pain	1
Verbal		
	Oriented and converses	5
	Disoriented but converses	4
	Inappropriate words	3
	Incomprehensible words	2
	Nonverbal	1

4. As has been emphasized throughout this text, the first priority in all patients is the airway and breathing. Unless the airway is secure, any further therapy will be futile. Patients with severe head injuries should be viewed as respiratory emergencies because of the high risk for developing airway complications.

There are essentially three options for securing the airway in the patient with severe head injury: orotracheal intubation, nasotracheal intubation, and cricothyroidotomy. Cricothyroidotomy should be performed only if orotracheal or nasotracheal intubation are contraindicated or attempts at intubation are unsuccessful. While nasotracheal intubation has its proponents, it does have inherent drawbacks when applied to the head injury patient. During nasotracheal intubation, the posterior pharynx is often irritated, which can induce vomiting. This not only increases the risk of aspiration but also causes an increase in the intracranial pressure. As a result, orotracheal intubation with rapid sequence induction is preferred in the patient with severe head injury. This involves the preintubation administration of medications.

As the patient is being preoxygenated with 100% oxygen and the cervical spine is stabilized, either an ultra short acting barbiturate, a benzodiazepine, or opioid analgesic should be administered. Barbiturates are useful because they not only produce adequate sedation but also increase cerebral perfusion by lowering the intracranial pressure. Their biggest drawback is that they are myocardial depressants and should not be utilized in the hypotensive patient. Benzodiazepines (e.g., midazolam or diazepam) provide sedation and an amnesic effect but have no effect on the intracranial pressure. Opioid analgesics (e.g., morphine, fentanyl) are readily reversible but can cause hypotension.

Intravenous lidocaine is also administered prior to intubation based on the premise that it blunts bronchospasm and tracheal irritation and an associated rise in intracranial pressure.

The next step is the administration of a paralytic agent. Succinylcholine (1.0 to 1.5 mg/kg) is a depolarizing agent which has traditionally been employed because of its rapid onset of action (60 seconds). Its greatest drawback is that it induces muscle fasciculations, but this effect can be countered by giving a "blocking dose" of pancuronium (0.01 mg/kg in the adult). Vercuronium, a rapid nondepolarizing agent, is now being utilized with increasing frequency.

After the paralytic agent is administered, cricoesophageal pressure (Sellick's maneuver) should be applied. Always assume the patient undergoing emergency intubation has a full stomach. Sellick's maneuver helps prevent aspiration and also assists with visualization of the vocal cords.

Once the patient is intubated and tube position confirmed, the patient should be hyperventilated. The goal is a $PaCO_2$ of approximately 25 mm Hg. By lowering the $PaCO_2$ to this level, the intracranial pressure can be safely, rapidly and reversibly lowered by inducing vasoconstriction of the arterioles (helping to decrease brain swelling). Caution against excessive hyperventilation needs to be exercised, as a $PaCO_2$ below 20 mm Hg has been associated with induction of brain tissue ischemia.

5. The primary goal of Emergency Department management of acute head trauma is to prevent secondary brain injury resulting from anoxia and decreased cerebral perfusion. The need for rapid and controlled airway management has already been discussed. Adequate oxygenation and ventilation are essential since hypoxia and hypercarbia can convert reversible brain injuries into irreversible injuries.

Hypotension also needs to be rapidly corrected—every attempt must be made to restore an adequate blood pressure (mean arterial pressure of 90 to 100 mm Hg). The converse is not true—attempts to decrease the blood pressure in the face of trauma can be disastrous. If the blood pressure remains consistently elevated, analgesics should be the first drug employed. It cannot be overstated that shock is almost never secondary to head injury until the terminal stage.

The gold standard for the diagnosis of focal lesions in head trauma is computed axial tomography (CAT). Indications for CAT include persistent altered level of consciousness, neurological deterioration, persistent neurological deficit, and clinical suspicion of a depressed skull fracture or basilar skull fracture. If a CAT scanner is not available, the patient should be transferred to another facility as soon as the patient is stabilized. Skull x-rays are only helpful in penetrating trauma or for evaluating depressed fractures.

Pharmacologic management of the head trauma patient needs to be individualized. Mannitol has traditionally been the first-line agent for lowering intracranial pressure, through its action as an osmotic diuretic. However, a rebound effect with increased bleeding has been associated with mannitol use, and therefore, its use should be restricted to patients who are undergoing a definitive study or surgery or appear to be herniating. Mannitol takes 20 to 30 minutes to take effect. Mannitol should not be administered to the hypovolemic patient.

Furosemide is also used to combat an elevated intracranial pressure. Besides decreasing total body water, it also decreases CSF production. When utilizing diuretic agents, it is important to monitor serum osmolality and replace fluids with isotonic solutions, as both hypoosmolality and hyperosmolality are harmful.

Other pharmacologic agents that have been employed in head trauma patients are corticosteroids, sedatives, paralytics, anticonvulsants, and vasopressors. Most authorities now agree that there is no proven benefit to steroid therapy for head trauma although they may be beneficial in spinal cord trauma. Sedatives and paralytics have already been discussed in airway management. The philosophy behind the use of anti-convulsants is that it is always better to prevent a seizure than to treat one. The anticonvulsant of choice is phenytoin. Anticonvulsants are particularly useful in cases of penetrating head trauma or head trauma with underlying brain lacerations, both of which are associated with a higher incidence of seizures. Recent interest has been expressed in the use of vasopressors, particularly dopamine, to increase the mean arterial pressure and consequently improve cerebral perfusion pressure.

Early neurosurgical consultation is essential in severe head trauma. In general, the prognosis of patients with severe head injuries is dependent on the time interval between the injury and treatment. For example, patients who have subdural hematomas and epidural hematomas evacuated under 4 hours do much better than those whose therapy is delayed beyond 4 hours.

An area of controversy is the use of burr holes for patients who demonstrate focal neurologic signs and evidence of herniation. Proponents of burr holes emphasize the time factor in evacuating a hematoma while opponents argue the high incidence of false localizing signs and difficulty not only in locating a hematoma but also in controlling bleeding.

Finally, there has been increasing interest in the use of Emergency Department intracranial pressure monitoring. Systems such as the Camino fiber optic system have simplified the monitoring process. The benefit of monitoring the intracranial pressure is that the physician can better determine when to start and stop treatment. A normal intracranial pressure is below 20 mm Hg, whereas an intracranial pressure greater than 30 mm Hg almost always leads to death unless treated and lowered.

<u>PEARLS</u>:

1. Fully 5 to 10% of patients with blunt head trauma have an associated cervical spine injury.

2. The prognosis for recovery worsens when elevated intracranial pressure is not treated within 4 hours with either surgical (mass lesion) or medical therapy (for diffuse axonal injury).

3. Patients with severe head injuries resulting from nonvehicular trauma such as falls or assault are much more likely to have surgically correctable lesions than victims of motor vehicle accidents.

4. The patient with a Glasgow Coma Score of 8 or less with unequal pupils and/or lateralizing deficits must be presumed to have a large focal lesion (e.g., epidural, subdural or intracerebral hematoma).

<u>PITFALLS</u>:

1. Hypotension is rarely due to a head injury in an adult except as a terminal event.

2. Do not assume a patient's decreased level of consciousness is due to alcohol or drugs.

3. Cushing's reflex (arterial hypertension and bradycardia in response to an elevated intracranial pressure) is a late and unreliable finding in acute head trauma.

4. One neurologic examination is not enough. The physician must continuously reassess neurologic status.

5. While a unilateral fixed dilated pupil is classically associated with contralateral hemiparesis, this is not always the case--the patient can have ipsilateral hemiparesis.

REFERENCES:

Ampel L, Hott KA, Sielaff AW, Sloan TB. An approach to airway management in the acutely head injured patient. J Emerg Med 1988;6:1-7.

Fink ME. Emergency management of the head injured patient. Emerg Med Clin North Am 1987;5:783-795.

Lillehei KO, Hoff JT. Advances in the management of closed head injury. Ann Emerg Med 1985;14:789-795.

Marshall LF, Smith RW, Shapiro HM. The outcome with aggressive treatment in severe head injuries. J Neurosurg 1979;50:20-30.

Roger JT. Risk management in emergency medicine. Dallas, TX: Emergency Medicine Foundation, 1985.

Springer MF, Baker FJ. Cranial burr hole decompression in the emergency department. Am J Emerg Med 1988;6:640-646.

NECK PAIN AFTER A FALL

Case 37:

A 78-year-old man was brought by a friend to the Emergency Department after he tripped on a rug in his home and fell and struck his forehead. He denied loss of consciousness. Initially, the patient stated he was unable to stand, but after lying on the floor for several minutes he was able to stand and call a neighbor for help. The patient's main concern was a burning feeling in his forearms and hands and mild neck pain. He denied visual disturbances, nausea, vomiting, or shortness of breath. His past medical history was significant for hypertension and arthritis in his back. His current medications were sulindac and verapamil. He denied recent use of alcohol.

On physical examination, the patient was noted to be alert and oriented, with a pulse of 50/minute and regular, blood pressure of 88/64 supine, and temperature of 98.1° F orally. The significant physical findings were an abrasion over the patient's forehead and slight tenderness to palpation of the upper cervical spine, although there was no stepoff or crepitus. In addition, the neurologic examination demonstrated bilateral weak hand grasps, 2/5 for the left hand and 3/5 for the right hand. The wrist extensors were 4/5 strength, while the proximal portions of the upper extremities demonstrated normal muscle strength. Gross functional motor strength of the lower extremities was normal (5/5). Additionally, the lower extremity reflexes were noted to be more brisk than the upper extremity reflexes. There was hyperesthesia over the forearms and hands; otherwise fine and sharp sensation were intact. The rectal tone was slightly diminished and the patient could not void spontaneously.

DIAGNOSTIC CLUES:

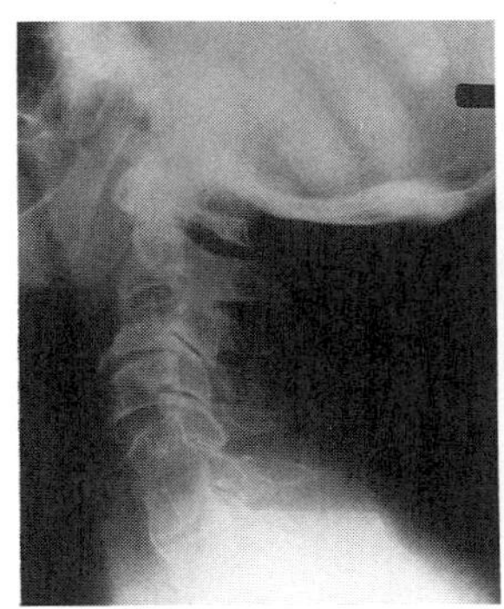

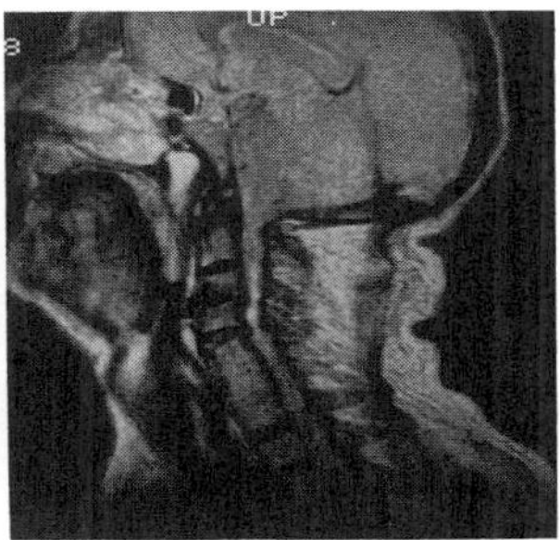

QUESTIONS:

1. What is the diagnosis?

2. When are cervical spine radiographs indicated? How many? When is CAT indicated?

3. Discuss "stable" versus unstable cervical spine fractures.

4. What are the neurological signs of spinal cord trauma?

5. What is the appropriate management of cervical spine injuries in the Emergency Department?

ANSWERS:

1. The roentgen diagnosis of this injury can be difficult unless the physician fully appreciates the history and clinical findings. At first glance, this x-ray appears relatively "normal" except for degenerative changes. However, when the clinical picture of a patient striking his forehead and being forced into hyperextension is combined with the neurologic findings, the suspicion of cervical spine injury increases. Radiographic signs of a hyperextension dislocation injury are an avulsion fracture of the anteroinferior aspect of the vertebra, prevertebral soft tissue swelling, widening of the disk space, and a vacuum defect (area of increased radiolucency) in the disk space. The findings in this patient of prevertebral soft tissue swelling and increased disk space are highly suggestive of a hyperextension dislocation injury.

How are the neurologic findings accounted for? The possibility of spinal cord injury in the elderly increases secondary to spondylosis and accompanying degenerative changes of the intervertebral disks and ligaments. In the scenario of hyperextension, the spinal cord becomes compressed between the arthritically enlarged vertebral ridge and the hypertrophied ligamentum flavum. The center of the cord is the most vulnerable area, and this explains why weakness is greater in the arms than in the legs and is worse in the hands than proximal upper extremities. The neuroanatomic basis for this is the orientation of the descending corticospinal tracts where those fibers innervating the arms and hands are located close to the center of the cord, while fibers to the legs are more lateral.

The most important step in the initial evaluation and diagnosis is to recognize that this is an incomplete or partial spinal cord injury, which has a much better prognosis than a complete cord lesion.

2. The routine ordering of cervical spine x-rays in any patient with significant blunt trauma stems from recommendations made throughout the trauma literature as well as concern for the highly disputable "asymptomatic" cervical spine injury. The importance of detecting cervical spine injury is obvious; nevertheless, cervical spine radiographs should be ordered with the same prudence as any other diagnostic study. In addition, physicians who labor under the illusion that normal cervical spine radiographs eliminate the possibility of cervical spine injury are likely to miss serious injuries.

The radiographic appearance of the spine after injury just represents its final or recoil position and is not always indicative of the forces generating the injury. The exact sensitivity and specificity of the routine three-view cervical spine series (cross table lateral, AP, and open mouth odontoid) depends on who is reading the films (e.g., experienced radiologist versus resident) and the technical accuracy of the films. However, they do serve as valuable screening tests when employed properly.

The first criterion for ordering x-rays should be the degree of alertness of the patient. Any patient who has sustained blunt trauma and is incapable of giving a good history (regardless of whether this is due to head injury, anoxia, alcohol, drugs, organic brain syndrome, or mental retardation) should have cervical spine x-rays. For the patient who can give a credible history and is responsive to the physical examination, the following are indications for radiographic studies: (1) patient complaining of neck pain, (2) tenderness to cervical spine palpation, (3) subjective or objective signs of spinal cord injury, or (4) major injury to some other body system that could possibly distract attention.

If the patient is completely alert and oriented with a clear mental status and none of the above four criteria are present, cervical spine films are not necessary. It is interesting that in one study over half of the patients who were determined not to need cervical spine x-rays subsequently had x-rays within 6 months of their injury.

One of the major pitfalls in evaluating cervical spine trauma is failure to adequately visualize the C6 to T1 region radiographically in adults. This area is particularly important when one considers that up to 30% of cervical injuries occur here in the adult patient. Reasons for difficulty in visualizing this region include patients who are muscular, obese or uncooperative and patients who have suffered trauma to the thorax, upper extremities or lower cervical spine. If gradual traction on the arms does not work, a swimmer's view should be attempted (this is done by extending the arm closest to the x-ray tube over the head, while the other arm remains at the side). If this is still inadequate, the next step is a CAT scan of this region.

CAT scan has replaced plain tomography as the definitive study in evaluating cervical spine injury. Its advantages over conventional tomography are that it is quicker, it requires less radiation, and there is no need for movement of the patient. CAT scan is optimal when utilized in conjunction with plain films; it better delineates the craniocervical junction, posterior elements, and the spinal cord and its soft tissue support. The role of MRI in acute cervical spine trauma is being expanded, as MRI delineates actual spinal cord involvement better than CAT.

Flexion-extension views are done under the supervision of a physician when the plain films are normal but the stability of the region is still in doubt. Flexion-extension views are contraindicated if there is obvious cervical spine instability or if a neurologic deficit is present.

Other views recommended in the literature include oblique and pillar plain radiographs. While these views may offer better definition of the injury, they do not add to the screening sensitivity of the three-view series. The most important guiding principle when ordering radiographic studies of the cervical spine is the spine should remain immobilized until the responsible physician is satisfied with the evaluation of the cervical spine.

3. When the clinician is faced with a potential injury to the cervical spine, two initial considerations are a fracture or dislocation and stability or instability of the injury. The stability of the spinal column is maintained by the bony skeleton (vertebrae) and the associated soft tissue structures (ligaments, joint capsules, and intervertebral disks). The cervical spine can be viewed as a two-column construction: the anterior column, consisting of the vertebral bodies, intervertebral disks, and the anterior and posterior longitudinal ligaments, while the posterior column is composed of the facets, apophyseal joints, pedicles, lamina, spinous processes, and intervening ligaments.

A mechanically unstable spine is one which is unable to maintain the normal anatomic relationships between the spinal segments when subjected to normal physiological loads. Such is the case if both the anterior and posterior columns are disrupted. If one column is disrupted the injury is said to be potentially unstable. The following list classifies common cervical injuries as mechanically stable or unstable:

Unstable

a. Bilateral facet dislocation
b. Flexion tear drop fractur
c. Hangman's fracture (traumatic spondylolisthesis C2)
d. Jefferson fracture (burst fracture of C1)
e. Hyperextension fracture/dislocation (stable in flexion, unstable in extension)

Stable

a. Simple wedge compression fracture
b. Posterior neural arch fracture of atlas
c. Pillar fracture
d. Clay shoulder's fracture (fractured spinous process)

Confusing the issue is the fact that mechanically stable injuries can result in spinal cord damage from fracture fragments, herniated disks, or spinal vascular compromise. The converse is also true; a lesion may be mechanically unstable, but neurologically stable. It is also important to recognize that vertebral injury need not be present for spinal cord injury to exist. Therefore, any injury which demonstrates neurologic impairment or radiographic abnormalities demonstrating instability (e.g., subluxation greater than 3.5 mm displacement or greater than 11 degrees angulation between the inferior aspects of adjacent vertebral bodies) should be treated as if the spine were at risk for further injury.

4. A careful neurologic examination is necessary both to differentiate complete from incomplete cord lesions and to establish a baseline for future evaluation of improvement or deterioration. A complete cord lesion is one in which there are no clinical signs of cord function below the level of injury, while incomplete lesions have some preservation of

cord function. The extent of neurologic examination is dictated by the patient's level of consciousness.

The basic neurologic examination for the patient who is alert and oriented begins with asking the patient to take a deep breath; this will allow the clinician to ascertain if both the intercostal and diaphragmatic muscles are functioning. Next, ask the patient to shrug his shoulders, testing C5. Follow this maneuver by flexion of the elbow to test C6, extension of the elbow for evaluation of C7, and hand grasp to test C8/T1 nerve function. Flexing the hips and raising the legs tests L2, L3 and L4, and wiggling the toes back and forth tests L5/S1. Anal sphincter tone is controlled by S2, S3 and S4.

Both light and sharp sensation should be tested, starting from abnormal and moving to normal. Conscious patients will often experience pain in the sensory dermatome corresponding to the level of injury. There is usually a relatively limited neurologic deficit with C1 and C2 injuries.

Clinical findings suggesting cervical spine injury in the unconscious patient include (1) flaccid areflexia, (2) diaphragmatic breathing, (3) response only to painful stimuli above the clavicles, (4) hypotension and bradycardia without any evidence of hypovolemic shock, (5) hyperthermia, and (6) priapism.

Perhaps the most important area to examine in the unconscious patient is the sacral region. Both the bulbocavernosus reflex and anal wink reflex are cord-mediated pathways. The bulbocavernosus reflex is elicited by either squeezing the base of the penis or vulva or tugging on a Foley catheter and observing for contraction of the anal sphincter. The anal wink reflex is brought about by applying a painful stimulus to the skin around the anus, resulting in contraction of the external anal sphincter.

5. A three-tiered approach to cervical spine trauma is necessary. The first priority, as always, is the ABC's. The second step is stabilization of the cervical spine, and the third phase is initiating treatment which may allow a greater chance for recovery. Respiratory insufficiency must be anticipated in patients with suspected cervical spinal cord injury. Trauma to the spinal cord can result in paralysis of the intercostal muscles or even phrenic nerve paralysis. The neck moves to some extent with both oro- or nasotracheal intubation. Therefore, if definitive airway management is indicated, someone must be assigned to immobilize the head and neck with in-line stabilization (not traction).

Hypotension in patients with cervical spine injuries can result from either hypovolemia secondary to other injuries or neurogenic shock from loss of sympathetic tone and resultant decrease in systemic vascular resistance, dilation of capacitance vessels, and unopposed parasympathetic stimulation of the heart. It is important to use caution when hydrating patients with suspected neurogenic shock, as pulmonary edema can result from overzealous fluid administration.

Ideally, resuscitation and stabilization of the cervical spine should be accomplished simultaneously. One of the major advances in prehospital care has been increased awareness of potential spinal cord injuries and the correct use of spinal immobilization techniques. It has been estimated that 10% of patients sustain further neurologic damage because of careless management on the part of prehospital and hospital personnel. Regardless of the position in which the cervical spine is found, it should be immobilized in a neutral supine position and splinted from the top of the head to the bottom of the buttocks.

The well-publicized results of the second National Acute Spinal Cord Injury Study appear to indicate that high dose corticosteroids are beneficial if given within 8 hours of the injury and continued over the next 24 hours. According to investigators, the benefits of high dose steroids were seen for all levels of severity, although the more severely injured patients improved less.

Treatment begins with a bolus of 30 mg/kg of methylprednisolone given over 15 minutes, then a 45-minute wait, followed by a 23-hour infusion at 5.4 mg/kg/hr. Patients with gunshot wounds were excluded from the study as were patients who had sustained other life-threatening injuries, pregnant females, children younger than 13 years old, and patients who either were diabetic, had severe peripheral vascular disease, had a systemic infection or had acute gastrointestinal bleeding.

Additionally, the aforementioned study showed no benefit in administering naloxone at the doses utilized (5.4 mg/kg bolus followed by a 4.0 mg/kg/hr infusion over 23 hours). Other experimental drugs and modalities that require future investigation include clonidine, thyrotropin releasing hormone, dimethyl sulfoxide, and local spinal cord cooling.

Decisions regarding definitive cervical spine immobilization should be left to the neurosurgeon who will assume care of the patient. The goal of a cervical spine traction apparatus (e.g., Gardner Well tongs) is to maintain the position of the unstable spine and to achieve reduction, if indicated, by applying counterweights in an incremental manner. However, traction should not be applied injudiciously, as it can also cause harm and is contraindicated in certain injuries (e.g., atlantooccipital and atlantoaxial injuries). The role of spinal cord decompression surgery is extremely controversial, with only two certain indications: (1) deteriorating neurologic status and (2) irreducible dislocations.

The emergency physician also needs to anticipate and treat complications of spinal cord injury. These include paralytic ileus, urinary retention, and hypothermia. Paralytic ileus can result in vomiting with consequent aspiration, and should be managed with a naso- or orogastric tube. Urinary retention is also commonly seen with spinal cord trauma; if the volume of urine in the bladder exceeds 500 cc, the detrusor muscle can become dysfunctional, resulting in delay of return of bladder function. It is therefore necessary to catheterize the patient who cannot spontaneously void. Hypothermia can result from the cutaneous vasodilation and subsequent heat loss associated with neurogenic shock. Adequate measures should be implemented to preserve a normal body temperature.

Patients with significant cervical spine injury should receive definitive management in a regional trauma center or spinal injury center.

PEARLS:

1. Think of the ABC'S when viewing cervical spine films:
   A = alignment
   B = bone (e.g., height and shape of vertebra)
   C = cartilage (disk spaces)
   S = soft tissue space (retropharyngeal and retrotracheal space)

2. Patients presenting with upper extremity paraplegia or quadriplegia with normal cervical spine x-rays should be suspected of having sustained a hyperextension injury.

3. When spinal curvature on x-ray is reversed from spasm alone, there will be a uniform transition over several segments. An abrupt transition focused at one position is almost always due to traumatic disruption.

4. Sparing of sensation in the sacral region may be the only sign of an incomplete cord lesion.

5. Over one-half of the patients with upper cervical spine injuries will have evidence of head or facial trauma.

PITFALLS:

1. The most common error is failure to visualize all seven cervical vertebra including C7 on T1. Almost 30% of adult injuries occur between C6 and T1.

2. Do not assume that absence of spinal injury on x-ray means there is no cervical spinal cord injury. It is possible to disrupt all the ligamentous structures between two adjacent vertebrae without any associated bony injury.

3. Remember to search for other fractures and/or dislocations after one fracture is found. Up to two-thirds of patients with vertebral fractures have two or more spinal column injuries. The presence of one injury of the spine does not preclude a second injury.

4. Do not use a rigid collar alone for initial spinal immobilization. In order to adequately immobilize the unstable spine, the patient should have the head splinted with sandbags or some other apparatus and be placed on a long spinal board.

REFERENCES:

Brackey MB, Shepard MJ, Collins WF, et al. A randomized controlled trial of methylprednisolone or naloxone in the treatment of acute spinal cord injury. N Engl J Med 1990;322:1405-1411.

Freemeyer B, Knopp R, Piche J, et al. Comparison of five-view and three-view cervical spine series in the evaluation of patients with cervical trauma. Ann Emerg Med 1989;18:818-821.

Harris JH, Edeiken-Monroe B. The radiology of acute cervical spine trauma 2nd ed. Baltimore: William & Wilkins, 1987.

McNamara RM, O'Brien MC, Davidheider S. Post-traumatic neck pain: a prospective and follow-up study. Ann Emerg Med 1988;17:906-911.

Ringenberg BJ, Fisher Ak, Urdaneta LF. Rational ordering of cervical spine radiographs following trauma. Ann Emerg Med 1988;17:748-796.

Scher AT. Hyperextension trauma in the elderly: an easily overlooked spinal injury. J Trauma 1983;23:1066-1068.

A YOUNG MAN WITH FLANK PAIN

Case 38:

A 38-year-old white male presented complaining of severe "crampy" pain in his right lower back for 3 hours. He had been in his usual state of health and quite active, including several hours of strenuous tennis earlier that day. The pain began while he was sitting down, was localized to his right flank, and radiated down into his groin. He described the quality of the pain as continuous with intermittent worsening, and the severity of the pain as "the worst of my life." He denied any previous episodes of pain.

He had vomited once since the onset of the pain, without hematemesis or coffee grounds. His last bowel movement was of normal consistency and color on the previous day; he denied any history of hematochezia or melena. There was no history of fever, dysuria, urinary frequency, urgency, or local trauma. His medical history was significant for mild hypertension for 5 years, controlled with propranolol 80 bid. He was on no other medications, denied any allergies, had a 10 pack/year smoking history but have quit 5 years earlier, drank one to two mixed drinks weekly, and denied use of any recreational drugs.

On physical examination, he was a well-developed, diaphoretic man writhing in pain on the stretcher. His blood pressure was 140/90, his pulse was 72/minute, his respiratory rate was 20/minute, and a rectal temperature was 99.6° F. His lungs were clear bilaterally. He had a normal S1 and S2, with an intermittent S4 and no murmurs or rubs. His abdomen was soft with moderate tenderness on his right anterior flank. His bowel sounds were normal. He had no hepatosplenomegaly or masses. Rectal examination revealed a normal-size, nontender prostate and heme-negative stool. His back was exquisitely tender to light percussion at the right costovertebral angle. His genital exam revealed no penile discharge and no scrotal swelling or tenderness. His extremities were not edematous. A complete neurologic exam was difficult due to the patient's discomfort, but his mental status as well as sensory and motor function were judged normal.

DIAGNOSTIC CLUE;

Urinalysis:

- pH 5.0
- Specific gravity 1.015
- Protein trace
- Glucose and ketones negative
- White cells 1-2/hpf
- Red blood cells 10-20/hpf
- Many crystals present

QUESTIONS:

1. What is the likely diagnosis of this patient's acute abdominal pain?

2. What points should be noted in the history?

3. What is the appropriate therapy?

4. What laboratory tests should be ordered?

5. Should this patient be warned to expect a recurrence of symptoms in the future?

ANSWERS:

1. Acute abdominal pain can be roughly diagnosed by quadrant, as diagrammed below.

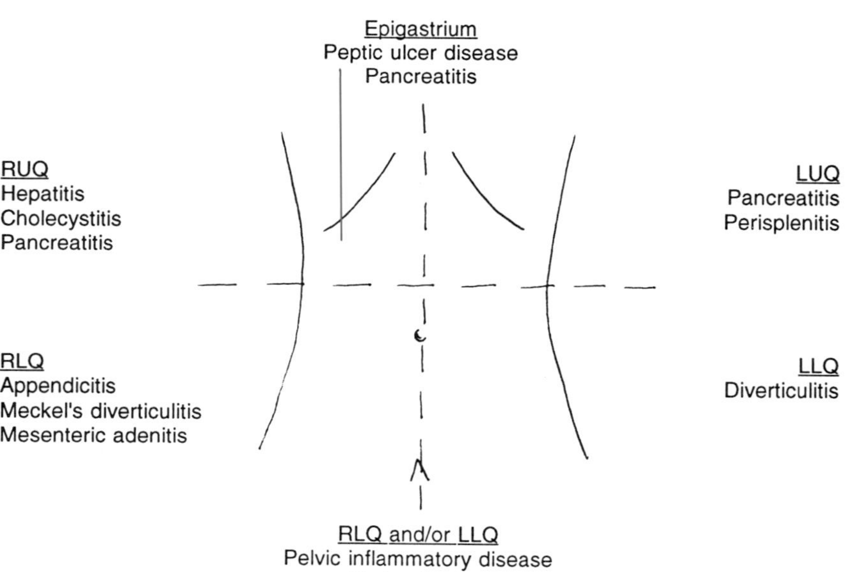

Back
Aortic aneurysm
Renal calculus
Choledocholithiasis
Pancreatitis

The pain described by this patient is severe, of sudden onset, and localized to the right flank with radiation to the groin. The diagnosis is renal colic until proven otherwise. Less likely possibilities include appendicitis, mesenteric adenitis, Meckel's diverticulitis, epididymitis, or pyelonephritis. His clinical examination is not suggestive of acute appendicitis, mesenteric adenitis, or Meckel's diverticulitis, particularly in view of the fact that the pain is predominantly localized to the costovertebral angle. His genital exam excludes the likelihood of epididymitis. Pyelonephritis can produce severe pain at the costovertebral angle; however, the onset is generally more gradual, is associated with a fever, and is accompanied by symptoms, of urinary tract infection and the pain is less intermittent.

Renal colic is a severe pain produced by partial or complete obstruction of the urinary outflow tract by one or more calculi, blood clots, or sloughed papillae. The severity of the pain has been compared to that of labor pain. Renal colic may be accompanied by hematuria, urgency, nausea, vomiting, or ileus.

Stones obstructing the renal pelvis and proximal ureter cause severe flank pain. As the stone passes downward, pain may radiate anteriorly around the abdomen to the testes, labia minora, or round ligament. Stones at the ureterovesical unction may produce symptoms mimicking cystitis or urethritis. High fever, diaphoresis, and chills are suggestive of concurrent pyelonephritis or urosepsis.

2. Key points in the history include the time course of events, pattern of pain, associated symptoms, personal and family history of calculi, and factors predisposing to papillary necrosis. A family history of calculi is found in inherited disorders, such as cystinuria, primary hyperoxaluria, and renal tubular acidosis. The patient should be questioned about conditions associated with renal lithiasis, such as hyperparathyroidism, hypercalcemia, enteric hyperoxaluria (associated with intestinal bypass procedures), gout, sarcoidosis, and infection.

Environmental factors play a role in the pathogenesis of renal calculi. Hot climates produce a higher incidence of stones, most likely as a result of increased evaporative loss from the skin and lungs. There is a seasonal increase in urinary calcium during summer months, possibly due to ultraviolet radiation stimulation of vitamin D synthesis. Patients who have larger adipose stores have increased perspiration to cope with heat dissipation, and they require more intake in order to maintain adequate urine volume, particularly during exertion. '

Low urine volume is an important risk factor. This can be caused by bowel disease with excess fluid loss, hyperhidrosis, self-imposed restriction of fluid intake by patients with urinary incontinence, or job-related restrictions which prevent ready access to toilet facilities.

Prolonged bedrest increases the propensity for renal stone formation, primarily by increasing calcium excretion. Hypercalciuria can be greater in younger individuals because of their increased bone turnover. Infection in the urine is also a risk factor for stone formation. Urea-splitting organisms promote struvite (triple phosphate stone) formation.

Medications may promote kidney stones, including vitamins A, C, and D; acetazolamide; ammonium chloride; protein supplements; calcium supplements; alkali; and antacids. These drugs may increase urinary calcium, such as excesses in vitamin D and ammonium chloride. They may change urinary pH and may alter citrate, such a ammonium chloride, alkali, and absorbable antacids. In addition, they may contain large amounts of calcium, such as calcium carbonate and calcium citrate. Some antacids produce calciuria by causing phosphate depletion.

3. Most renal calculi are less than 4 to 5 mm in size and will pass spontaneously. They can be managed conservatively with analgesics such as meperidine 75 to 100 mg IM, nonsteroidal antiinflammatory drugs such as indomethacin (which can be given as a suppository), or Toradol and generous hydration (at least 200 cc/hour either PO or IV). Care must be taken with patients who cannot tolerate large quantities of intravenous fluids.

If the patient's pain is controlled with this therapy in the Emergency Department, he can be sent home with oral analgesics such as oxycodone/acetaminophen (Percocet) for several days. The patient should be instructed to maintain optimal hydration and to strain all urine for recovery of calculi. The patient should be made to understand the necessity of bringing any strained stones to a physician for analysis. A follow-up appointment should be made within a week.

The following patients will need to be admitted to the hospital for further therapy:

a. Presence of infection or fever greater than 101° F
b. Refractor pain
c. Sufficient nausea and vomiting to prevent adequate fluid intake or oral analgesics at home
d. Patients with only one kidney or a transplanted kidney

4. Metabolically speaking, there are four causes of kidney stone disease: primary hypercalciuria, hyperoxaluria, hypocitraturia, and hyperuricosuria. Primary hypercalciuria can be of three types: absorptive, renal, or resorptive. Absorptive hypercalciuria results from increased calcium absorption from the small intestine and accounts for about 50% of all cases of renal calculi disease. Renal hypercalciuria is the result of decreased tubular reabsorption of calcium. Resorptive hypercalciuria usually occurs because of increased endogenous production of parathyroid hormone by a parathyroid adenoma.

Hyperoxaluria is seen in children as the result of enzyme disorders and increased hepatic production of oxalate. In adults, hyperoxaluria is commonly caused by fat malabsorption due to inflammatory bowel disease, ileal resection, jejunoileal bypass for obesity, or chronic biliary or pancreatic disease. Other causes include diet high in leafy green vegetables, colas, and chocolate; excessive intake of vitamin C; methoxyflurane anesthesia; and ethylene glycol intoxication.

Hypocitraturia can be caused by distal renal tubular acidosis, chronic diarrheal states, hydrochlorothiazide therapy, hypokalemia, urinary tract infection, and idiopathic calcium oxalate nephrolithiasis. The uric acid stones of hypocitraturia as pH-dependent, with a decrease in pH resulting in an increase in formation of cystine and uric acid crystals.

Hyperuricosuria is cause by primary gout, severe dehydration, chronic diarrheal states, myeloproliferative syndromes, and chemotherapy. The struvite (magnesium ammonium phosphate) stones that result are formed by urea-splitting bacteria such as Proteus species. Such bacteria produce ammonia and an alkaline pH, thus promoting struvite precipitation.

The patient who presents to the Emergency Department with a first renal calculus should have a blood chemistry analysis with determination of serum calcium, chloride, phosphorus, uric acid, creatinine, and carbon dioxide level and have a complete blood count. Although a slight elevation may occur in the white blood cell count with renal colic, a significant elevation (over 15,000) is highly suggestive of concomitant infection. A urine sample must be examined for crystals and blood as well as to check pH. The presence of pyuria indicates the need for a urine culture. If a stone is passed and collected, x-ray crystallographic analysis should be requested.

A KUB film should always be obtained if renal colic is suspected. Over 80% of calcium (calcium phosphate, calcium oxalate, struvite) stones are radiopaque and will be evident on plain film. Uric acid stones, sloughed papillae, and blood clots will not be visualized. It is occasionally necessary to obtain films in the right or left posterior oblique or lateral positions to define further calcified densities that are not definitely calculi. An intravenous pyelogram should be obtained in order to rule out residual obstruction or the presence of other stones. Indications for an emergency intravenous pyelogram include the following:

a. Inability to distinguish between renal colic, appendicitis, and cholecystitis
b. Necessity of ruling out an impacted stone with infection behind the stone in patients with colic and fever
c. Persistent hematuria and colic

patients with recurrent stone disease require a more extensive laboratory evaluation in addition to the emergency diagnostic studies delineated above. The bulk of these studies can be completed on an outpatient basis and are not relevant to emergency management of renal colic.

5. Between 1 and 10% of the population will have a kidney stone at some time in their lives, and the recurrence rate is 50 to 70%. The patient should be advised of the risk of recurrence and the steps he should take to minimize the risk of recurrence. Attention to good hydration is key, particularly after meals and exercise, when the urine solute load is highest. Follow-up by a physician is essential, with a repeat KUB recommended in approximately 6 months to monitor for recurrent calcified stone formation.

PEARLS:

1. In contrast to the patient with peritoneal pain who lies very still, the patient with renal colic is usually thrashing about trying to find a comfortable position.

2. The renal colic patient should be sent home with a stack of gauze and instructed to urinate through the gauze in order to effectively strain the urine and recover stones.

PITFALLS:

1. Urinalysis for identification of crystal types is generally not helpful. Cystine and struvite crystals provide a clue to the type of stone material, but other crystals are often seen in the nonstone-forming patients, particularly in urine samples studied at room temperature.

2. Low-grade fever may be attributed to renal colic alone, but a high-grade fever should be presumed to indicate infection.

3. Be wary of diagnosing nephrolithiasis in a patient over 50 years of age with a first episode of renal colic. The presentation of abdominal aortic aneurysm can mimic that of a kidney stone and must be excluded.

REFERENCES:

Hugosson J, Grenabo L, Hedelin H, et al. Bacteriology of upper urinary tract stones. J Urol 1990;143(5):965-968.

Laporte J, Baum N. Kidney stones. How to identify the cause and prevent recurrence. Postgrad Med 1990; 87(5):219-223, 226.

Smith I. Urography during renal colic. Br J Surg 1986;53(2):93-102.

Smith JJ 3d, Hollowell JG, Roth RA. Multimodality treatment of complex renal calculi. J Urol 1990;143(5):891-894.

Uribarri J, Oh MS, Carroll HJ. The first kidney stone. Ann Int Med 1989;111:1006-1009.

INDEX